DASH DIET COOKBOOK

A culinary approach to reduce hypertension

Contents

PART 1:

EVERYTHING YOU NEED TO KNOW ABOUT DASH DIET

This easy-to-read and comprehensive cookbook is written for all the individuals and beginners who lead busy and on-the-go lifestyles and struggle to find the time to prepare a wholesome meal plan that follows the guidelines of the DASH Diet, with an approach to provide a comprehensive resource that not only educates readers about the DASH Diet but also offers practical solutions for incorporating it into their daily lives.

The centerpiece of this cookbook is a collection of DASH Diet recipes crafted to streamline meal preparation and ensure an easy transition to healthier eating habits. Each recipe has been tested and proven to enhance health outcomes, providing a delicious yet nutritious dining experience. Despite their lower calorie and fat content, all the recipes are designed to satisfy and energize dieters. This cookbook is perfect for homemakers and people with hypertension seeking to maintain a balanced diet without sacrificing flavor or satiety.

Whether you need help finding time for meal planning, are unsure how to adhere to the DASH Diet guidelines or are simply looking to improve your overall health and fitness, this cookbook is just for you.

From managing high blood pressure and reducing hypertension to boosting physical fitness and shedding unwanted pounds, the recipes, tips, tricks, shopping lists, and meal plans in this cookbook offer a holistic approach to hypertension-free living.

If you are positive and motivated to protect your health and reduce the onset of chronic conditions like high blood pressure, then this book is your ultimate companion. we hope this cookbook guides you on the road to a healthy and happy life.

Your journey is better if you begin here, and I am confident that the insights and recipes shared in this book will prove invaluable in your quest for vitality and well-being.

Introduction

As by its name, this cookbook is all about experiencing the remarkable DASH Diet and availing its benefits through a culinary approach. In today's modern society, where everyone is overwhelmed with unnecessary and fluff information regarding various dietary plans, the DASH Diet stands out as the tower of health and vitality.

The basic purpose of writing this cookbook is to help people between the ages of 30-60 understand the effective use of sodium in their meals by choosing alternatives for controlling their hypertension.

As we get older, the most common health issue faced by most of us is high blood pressure, and what makes the overall situation more threatening is the improper treatment that later changes into life-threatening issues like heart attack, strokes, and kidney failure. So, if you are a middle-aged person suffering from hypertension, then this book is for you. But age is just a number; beginners or sufferers can use this book.

The DASH Diet approaches your daily eating habits in such a way that prevents high blood pressure. The DASH Diet also helps to increase the metabolism rate. The DASH Diet incorporates fruits, vegetables, less fat, and low-sodium food.

This book's primary focus is middle-aged people suffering from hypertension who lack time to address the problem or prepare a meal that helps them control this illness. It contains basic information about the DASH Diet, its health benefits, and why it is good for the health and overall fitness of beginners, the whole family, and especially middle-aged men and women.

For most of us, the word "Diet" seems frustrating, while thinking of ditching certain favorite food items seems unappealing. It is not the case with the DASH Diet, as it is not a magical elixir that promises quick results in a shorter time. Unlikely, it is a lifestyle to follow to cure recurring health conditions.

With great pride, we have introduced you to this comprehensive cookbook with profound inside guidance. It helps everyone promote a healthy and fit lifestyle through meals and collections of recipes that help control hypertension and boost a healthy metabolism. The primary objective of writing this cookbook is to educate beginners, senior citizens, people with busy lifestyles, homemakers, and health enthusiasts about the DASH Diet.

This cookbook helps beginners kick start their journey and transform their busy lifestyle by trying delicious and healthy home-cooked recipes concerning their high blood pressure, heart health, and weight loss. So, if you want to taste home-cooked dishes that are nutritious, cheap, and have widely available ingredients, then this cookbook is just for you.

In today's hectic society, most people are so busy that they eat junk food and order takeaway. Lacking time to prepare home-cooked meals makes them indulge in unhealthy eating habits. Junk food significantly contributes to obesity and the development of hypertension, as the high sodium content in junk and processed food leads to water retention in the body, thus causing increased blood volume and raising blood pressure. It also lacks essential nutrients like vitamins, minerals, protein, and fiber.

Excessive calorie intake leads to weight gain, which becomes a risk factor for hypertension. The increase in body fat because of obesity, especially around the abdomen, increases the release of hormones and inflammatory substances inside the body that disturb the regulation of blood pressure. Also, obesity is associated with insulin resistance and metabolic syndromes, which further contribute to hypertension.

We all know that all junk foods are high in Tran's fats, and saturated fat increases LDL and reduces HDL cholesterol; thus, it increases and contributes to the fatty plaque that builds inside the arteries and causes blood pressure to rise. The hypertension development that, when untreated, damages the blood vessels and interferes with the normal function of the cardiovascular system.

The primary objective behind writing this cookbook is to clarify the significance of sodium management in combating high blood pressure (BP) and hypertension. In today's world, a considerable number of individuals struggle with issues such as excess weight, elevated BP, and hypertension. Accumulating the challenge is the potential progression of these conditions into severe health complications, including strokes, kidney failure, and heart attacks, if left untreated and unmanaged. Recognizing this urgent need, the DASH Diet emerges as a proactive approach to dietary habits that not only lessen the risk of high blood pressure and hypertension but also boost the metabolism. Moreover, the DASH Diet plan extends its benefits to individuals seeking to shed unwanted weight gain by indulging in the healthy consumption of fruits, vegetables, and low-fat, low-sodium products.

In addition to unveiling the principles of the DASH Diet, this book is consistent with an array of delectable recipes covering a variety of breakfast, lunch, dinner, snacks, and beverages. These culinary creations are carefully prepared to satisfy your palate and support your efforts to maintain optimal BP levels and ward off hypertension. Furthermore, accompanying these recipes are simple yet effective guidelines that facilitate the seamless integration of the DASH Diet into your daily meal planning.

I invite you to dive into the sea of information and culinary inspiration in this cookbook, which holds the key to lowering high blood pressure and hypertension and fostering a metabolism that thrives on wholesome nutrition.

In today's fast-paced world, where processed foods and unhealthy eating habits have become common, the DASH Diet offers a refreshing alternative and a return to the basics of wholesome, nourishing foods that promote optimal health.

Developed by researchers at the National Institutes of Health (NIH), the DASH Diet emphasizes consuming vegetables, grains, fruits, seeds, lean proteins, and low-fat dairy products while limiting sodium, saturated fats, and added sugars. Its primary focus is to prevent and manage hypertension, or high blood pressure, a condition that affects millions of people worldwide and is a significant and primary factor for stroke, heart disease, and other serious health issues.

As you start your DASH Diet journey with the help of this cookbook, you'll discover a treasure of delicious and nutritious recipes designed to tantalize your taste buds while nourishing your brain and body.

From smoothies bursting with color and flavor to hearty dinners that warm the soul, each dish carefully aligns with the DASH Diet protocols and makes healthy eating a joyous and satisfying experience.

But the DASH Diet is not limited to just recipes; it's a holistic approach to wellness that encompasses mindful eating, regular physical activity, and a supportive community, and this is what this cookbook's primary aim is. In this cookbook, you'll find culinary inspiration, practical tips for meal planning, grocery shopping, dining out, and insights into the science behind the DASH Diet and its proven health benefits. Whether you're a busy housewife, a senior adult suffering hypertension, or a naïve in the kitchen, whether you're seeking to improve your health or broaden your culinary skills, there's something here for everyone.

This cookbook is written with the belief that food is not just fuel for the body but also nourishment for the soul—a source of joy, connection, and creativity. In that spirit, it invites you to embrace the DASH Diet not as a restrictive regimen but as a celebration of nature's abundance and variety of wholesome foods. Let these recipes guide you as you explore new flavors, experiment with fresh ingredients, and discover the transformative power of healthy eating.

This book is a trusted companion for better health and well-being. May each meal you prepare from these pages bring you closer to the aims and goals and inspire you to live your best life—one delicious bite at a time. Cheers to a future filled with vitality, happiness, and good health.

Once again, I express my appreciation for selecting this book, and I sincerely hope you find it both informative and enjoyable. Embrace the DASH Diet and embark on a transformative journey toward a healthier, happier you!

CHAPTER NO 1:
What Is Dash Diet?

Welcome to DASH Diet (Dietary Approach to Lower Blood Pressure and Reduce Hypertension). As per the title of this chapter, you will be given a proper introduction to the DASH Diet and guidelines for lowering high-bold pressure. The DASH Diet is a diet plan that makes you legitimately sacrifice taste.

Currently, more than 50 million people in the U.S.A. and more than a billion people around the world are suffering from hypertension. We humans eat food to survive, but the choices we make not only reflect our culture, values, and norms but also affect our health.

In today's modern society, bad eating habits lead to many recurring health issues and illnesses that likely create an urge to go back to the simple lifestyle with much more concentration on home-cooked meals that provide solutions or culinary approval to overcome or reduce the effect or symptom of illness.

It has been proven that a dietary approach could be adapted to control high blood flow and hypertension.

Moreover, when we see our recurring health condition, our doctors usually recommend that we follow a "DASH Diet." So, it is essential to understand this diet plan clearly.

Definition of the DASH Diet

This diet stands for Dietary Approaches to Cure Hypertension. This diet is designed to help lower or prevent high blood pressure (hypertension) by emphasizing the consumption of nutrient-rich foods that are high in potassium, calcium, fiber, and magnesium and low in sodium. It is a proven diet plan to support heart health and reduce blood pressure levels.

The DASH Diet primarily focuses on lowering blood pressure and maintaining a flexible, healthy weight. Its protocols involve reducing saturated fat and cholesterol by consuming less fat and more fruits and vegetables.

The plan incorporates low-fat dairy products, seeds, nuts, whole grains, beans, fish, and poultry. It limited salt, added sugar, beverages, processed food items, and red meat consumption.

Reducing salt intake in daily meals has a more significant impact on health, as excessive salt consumption causes hypertension, high blood pressure, kidney disease, heart failure, and cirrhosis.

It is said and cleared in the Dietary Guidelines for Americans (2010) that the sodium intake should not exceed 1500 mg daily. The DASH Diet is recommended for people with kidney diseases, high blood pressure, diabetes, African Americans, and older and middle-aged adults. Embracing the DASH Diet can initiate a healthier lifestyle.

Critical Aspects of the DASH Diet

Blood Pressure Management: The DASH Diet prioritizes flexibly lowering high blood pressure and maintaining healthy levels.

Low Saturated Fat and Cholesterol: The plan emphasizes consuming foods low in saturated fat and cholesterol.

Focus on Fruits and Vegetables: A primary emphasis is placed on incorporating a variety of fruits and vegetables into meals.

Inclusion of Low-Fat Dairy Products: The diet includes dairy products that are low in fat to support overall health.

Rich Whole Grains and Lean Proteins: Whole grains, beans, seeds, nuts, fish, and poultry are encouraged as sources of essential nutrients.

Limited Sodium, Added Sugar, and Red Meat: The DASH Diet advocates for reduced salt intake, added sugars, beverages, and red meat.

Health Impact of Lowering Salt Intake: Decreasing salt intake can significantly impact health by reducing the risk of hypertension, high blood pressure, kidney disease, heart failure, and cirrhosis.

Recommended Sodium Intake: According to the "Dietary Guidelines for Americans, 2010," daily sodium intake should not exceed 1500 mg.

Targeted Recommendations: The DASH Diet is recommended for individuals with kidney diseases, high blood pressure, diabetes, African Americans, and older and middle-aged adults.

Lifestyle Improvement: Embracing the DASH Diet can initiate a healthier lifestyle and promote overall well-being.

Start a Better Lifestyle with the DASH Diet

Based on the same advice elders used to give, " to eat veggies, fruit, and drink milk daily," the DASH Diet protocols approach the same to stop hypertension. Organic, fresh, and seasonal fruits and vegetables are incorporated into our recipe. Our goal is to avoid salt substitutes and instead utilize herbs and spices that impart a salty flavor to the meal, reducing the need for additional salt. Before beginning the cooking process, it is essential to understand the daily nutrient goals outlined in the DASH Diet.

The information is for a 2,000-calorie DASH Diet Eating Plan.
- Fat (Total)   27% of calories
- Fat (Saturated) 6% of calories
- Carbohydrates   55% of calories
- Protein   18% of calories
- Cholesterol   150 mg
- Potassium   4700 mg*

- Sodium   2300 mg
- Calcium 1,250 mg
- Magnesium   500 mg

Selecting the right ingredients is crucial as they significantly impact a recipe's fat, potassium, sugar, or sodium levels.

To reduce sodium intake, choose salt-free or low-sodium versions of products like beans, bouillon, or broth. It's important to carefully read labels before proceeding with cooking.

Let's embark on the DASH Diet journey, which promises to improve your health and happiness by lowering blood pressure and eliminating hypertension. You'll feel more energetic and content and may even shed some extra pounds and cultivate a strong desire for transformation.

Consult Your Physician Before Following The Diet

If you are already taking any hypertension medicines, then never discontinue any medication without medical guidance.
Regularly visit your doctor during the diet to monitor blood pressure.
Note that individual responses to diet plans may vary; for instance, individuals with kidney problems or other health issues may not experience the full benefits of the diet.

History and Origin of the DASH Diet

High blood pressure is one of the fastest and most widely spreading health conditions that affect about one-third of the population in the United States. A blood pressure reading above 145 /90 mmHg is considered to be high blood pressure. The first number, 140, is systolic blood pressure, extended by the blood against the artery while the heart is contracted. The bottom number 90 is considered to be diastolic blood pressure. This diastolic blood pressure is considered to be in the arteries while the heart is relaxing or between heartbeats. The primary concern was that hypertension patients had a greater risk of developing heart diseases, stroke, and kidney problems. High pressure is a silent silence that usually shows no symptoms or warning signs at the start.

The publication in the New England General of Medicines in 1977 was the first study conducted by the National Heart, Lung, and Blood Institute. This study looks at the effects of a diet rich in potassium, magnesium, and calcium on high blood pressure without any supplement.

The study was conducted on 459 adults with and without high blood pressure. The parameters were set that the systolic blood pressure had to be less than 160 mmHg and diastolic should be between 80 to 95 mmHg.

Half of the participants in the study were women, and 60% were African Americans. Thus, three eating plans were created and compared. The first diet plan was high in fat, with approximately 37% of the calories incorporated in fats; the diet does not focus on fruits and vegetables. In this typical American diet, fruit and vegetable consumption was deficient.

The second diet was American but based on fruit and vegetable consumption. The third diet plan was rich in fruits and vegetables and low in dietary food and fat (less than 30% calories). This third diet has 4700 mg of potassium, 500mg of magnesium, and 1240 mg of calcium per 2000 calories.

However, all three diet plans contain equal amounts of sodium, almost 3000 mg daily, equivalent to 7 grams of salt. The seven grams of salt intake was almost 20% below the average intake for adults in the United States, according to the current salt recommendation of 4 to 5 grams daily. The general calorie intake was according to the participant's weight.

The third diet plan then knowingly became the DASH Diet in the future. Reducing and eliminating salt intake and weight loss were the key reasons for any change in blood pressure. The meals for each participant were prepared in one Central kitchen to increase compliance with the diet.

The results show that the increased fruit and vegetable diet and DASH Diet plan lowered the blood pressure, but the DASH Diet was the most effective.

Participants who did not have high pressure reduced their systolic pressure by six mmHg and diastolic by three mmHg.

However, the results were even much better for the patients who were suffering from hypertension. For the patient with hypertension, the DASH Diet recorded the drop in their systolic and diastolic pressures almost double; the drops in systolic and diastolic were nearly 11 mmHg and 6 mmHg.

These clinical studies proved that the DASH Diet appears to lower and reduce blood pressure similarly to that seen with a single blood pressure medicine.

The DASH Diet showed results within two weeks of starting it, comparable to treatment by medication. This was continued throughout the trial. Thus, the prosecution proves calcium and magnesium are essential factors affecting blood pressure rather than sodium alone.

Recognition and Adoption

The DASH Diet gained recognition for its effectiveness in lowering high blood pressure and improving heart and cardiovascular health. It has been endorsed by various health organizations, including the American Heart Association (AHA) and the Dietary Guidelines for Americans.

Further Research and Modifications

Since its inception, further research has been conducted to refine the DASH Diet recommendations and explore its potential benefits for other health conditions, such as weight management, diabetes, and metabolic syndrome.

Overall, the DASH Diet remains a widely recommended dietary pattern for promoting heart health and managing hypertension, with its roots firmly grounded in scientific research and evidence-based practice.

Considerations in Clinical Practice

Gradually increase fiber intake to prevent gastrointestinal discomfort like bloating or gas. When customizing the DASH Diet, account for individual food allergies and intolerances (e.g., lactose intolerance). While the DASH Diet promotes overall health, it may not encompass every nutritious food. For instance, avocados are not typically included in DASH guidelines. Additionally, some foods within recommended categories, such as pretzels categorized as grains, may lack fiber and essential nutrients.
 Be mindful that individuals may have varying tolerances to salt restrictions. Gradually reducing daily salt intake could be beneficial to accommodate individual preferences and needs.

Consider integrating DASH Diet recommendations with complementary dietary approaches, such as the Mediterranean Diet, which also boasts substantial evidence supporting its efficacy.

Currently, over 1 billion individuals worldwide are struggling with hypertension. The correlation between elevated blood pressure and cardiovascular disease remains consistently significant. Individuals with hypertension face significantly heightened risks of experiencing heart attacks. To mitigate and manage the impacts of hypertension, the American National Institutes of Health (NIH) unveiled the DASH Diet regimen in 1992. Since its inception, the DASH Diet has emerged as a famous, successful, well-recognized, and productive approach stemming from NIH-funded research endeavors. For those struggling with hypertension, adopting the DASH Diet plan is strongly advised to preserve physical well-being.

CHAPTER 2:
Benefits of the DASH Diet

How Does DASH Diet Work?

As we age, we experience many health issues like muscle fatigue, lack of energy, and other illnesses. Many times, our recurring health issues put us on various prescriptions and treatment courses.

High blood pressure is a common and highly spreading issue for older people because of cardiovascular changes with aging. To reduce and cure hypertension, we recommend you follow a DASH Diet, a proven diet plan that helps reduce high blood pressure. The DASH Diet incorporates low-fat, low-sodium, and balanced ingredients that reduce hypertension. The focus is on containing low-sodium food items and, if possible, eliminating sodium from the meal. Now, your mind starts to think about whether sodium is that bad. So, let's get the answer.
What Is Sodium?

Sodium is a very distinctive element with a unique taste. Salt is not just sodium alone. The salt we consume is made from sodium and chloride. Salt and sodium are different. The salt we consume daily is beneficial, but to some extent, as excess can harm the body and brain. It's been recommended that all hypertension patients stay away from sodium or salt.

How Does Sodium Affect The Human Body?

About 0.9 percent of our body is sodium chloride. Sodium is essential as it helps maintain suitable electrolytes and cell function.
Sodium helps manage the following:

- Control the blood pressure level
- Helps in muscle contraction
- Balance the overall pH level
- Keep the body Hydrated
- Helps in effective nerve system transmission
- Help get rid of low blood pressure

Almost all the food items contain some quantity of natural sodium in them. For example, beef, celery, and milk contain sodium. Even natural water also contains sodium. Some foods contain excess sodium, like canned food and processed food items. We can incorporate sodium in our meals in three ways:

- Eating the food that contains it
- Using table salt
- Using natural sources
- Disadvantage of High Sodium Intake

Taking a lot of sodium can negatively affect a person's health. It is because it disturbs the body's fluid balance and controls the blood pressure line. These are some of the demerits mentioned above:

High Blood Pressure (also known as hypertension)

Sodium plays a vital role in controlling one's blood pressure. When sodium intake is high, the body may retain excess water, increasing blood volume and pressure on artery walls. This may eventually lead to hypertension, which is a major risk factor for serious diseases like heart attack, stroke, or other cardiovascular complications that develop over time.

Diseases of the Kidneys

The kidneys are important organs because they help maintain body salt balance. A large sodium intake stresses these organs since an increased workload is needed to eliminate excessive sodium from the bloodstream. It might eventually damage the kidneys over time and increase the chances of acquiring renal disorders like chronic kidney disease or kidney stones.

Atherosclerosis:

Atherosclerosis is a disorder that is characterized by the accumulation of plaque in the arteries. Excessive consumption of sodium can lead to the development of atherosclerosis, which can lead to a heart attack. Because of this narrowing of the arteries, blood flow to the heart might be restricted, increasing the chance of having a heart attack. This is especially true for people who have other risk factors, such as the presence of high cholesterol or diabetes.

Heart Failure

Consuming a high amount of salt can make heart failure worse by causing the body to retain fluid, resulting in swelling (edema) and putting additional strain on the heart. When persons who already have cardiac issues are exposed to excessive sodium, it can make their symptoms worse and increase the likelihood that they will experience bouts of heart failure.

Cirrhosis

It is a late-stage liver fibrosis caused by a variety liver diseases and ailments, including hepatitis and chronic alcoholism. Cirrhosis is a very life-threatening condition that affects the liver. A high sodium intake can make fluid retention worse in those who have cirrhosis, which can result in consequences such as ascites and more damage to the liver.

How Excess Sodium Cause Hypertension?

Consuming sodium interacts with potassium in your body to regulate the balance of acids in your blood cells. This interaction can lead to high blood pressure and decreased levels of calcium and magnesium in the body. Dehydration can further exacerbate this by causing potassium depletion and tissue damage.

For individuals with hypertension, it's advised to limit sodium intake to 1500 mg per day. However, athletes and those engaging in prolonged physical activity may need a higher sodium intake due to increased salt loss through sweating.

Part 2:

Recipes

CHAPTER 5:
10 BREAKFAST

Kiwi and Green Apple Smoothie

Ingredients:
- 1 kiwi, peeled
- 1/2 green apple, chopped
- 1/2 cup fat-free Greek yogurt
- 1/2 cup unsweetened almond milk
- 1/2 teaspoon chia seeds

 Easy

 0 minutes

 1

 5 minutes

 5 minutes

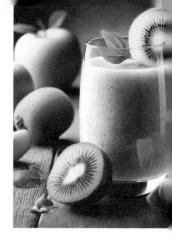

Nutritional Values per Serving:
Calories: Approx. 190
Total Fat: 2g (3%)
Saturated Fat: 0g (0%)
Cholesterol: 0mg (0%)
Sodium: 95mg (4%)
Total Carbohydrates: 35g (13%)
Dietary Fiber: 5g (18%)
Total Sugars: 24g
Protein: 10g

Directions:
1. Prepare all ingredients: peel the kiwi, chop the green apple.
2. Place the kiwi, green apple, Greek yogurt, almond milk, and chia seeds in a blender.
3. Blend for about 30-60 seconds or until the mixture is smooth and homogeneous.
4. Pour the smoothie into a glass and, if desired, add some ice cubes for a more refreshing effect.
5. Serve immediately and enjoy an energizing and nutritious drink.

Oats and Banana Pancakes

Ingredients:
- 1 cup rolled oats
- 1 ripe banana, mashed
- 2 eggs
- 1/2 cup almond milk
- 1 teaspoon baking powder
- 1/2 teaspoon cinnamon

 Simple

 15 minutes

 2

 10-12 minutes

 30 minutes

Nutritional Values per Serving:
Calories   545
% Daily Value*
Total Fat 19.8g   25%
Saturated Fat 9.1g   46%
Cholesterol 372mg   124%
Sodium 195mg   8%
Total Carbohydrate 91g   33%
Dietary Fiber 21.3g   76%
Total Sugars 8.8g
Protein 21.3g

Directions:
1. Take a high-speed blender and add rolled oats to it
2. Pulse the blender until the oats have a flour-like consistency.
3. In a mixing bowl, combine eggs, mashed bananas, cinnamon, baking powder, and almond milk.
4. Use a hand beater to combine all the things well together.
5. Slowly add the oat flour to the wet ingredients, stirring it until it combined well.
6. Heat a medium skillet over medium flame.
7. You can use a grill as well if you like,
8. Pour the 1/4 cup of the pancake batter onto the skillet.
9. Let it cook for 2-3 minutes until bubbles form on the surface.
10. Then flip the pancakes and cook from the other side for 2-3 minutes.
11. Repeat until all the batter for pancakes is consumed.
12. Once done, serve it with your favorite toppings, such as sliced strawberries, bananas, or a sprinkle of cinnamon.

Baked Vegetable Omelets

Ingredients:

- 4 organic eggs, whisked
- 1/4 cup reduced-fat milk or almond milk
- 1 cup fresh spinach, chopped
- 1/2 cup cherry tomatoes, halved
- 1/4 cup bell peppers, diced (any color)
- 1/4 cup onion, diced
- 1/4 cup zucchini, diced

Nutritional Values per Serving:

Calories   456
% Daily Value*

Total Fat 37.4g   48%

Saturated Fat 7.9g   40%

Cholesterol 372mg   124%

Sodium 173mg   8%

Total Carbohydrate 20.1g   7%

Dietary Fiber 7.8g   28%

Total Sugars 2.3g

Protein 16.5g

      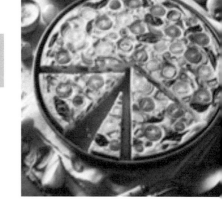

Simple   15 minutes   4

20-25 minutes   35-40minutes

Directions:

1. Before starting the cooking, preheat the oven to 375 degrees F for a few minutes.
2. Take a large mixing bowl and crack eggs in it.
3. Whisk the eggs and add milk.
4. Whisk it well.
5. Pour half of egg mixture into a non-stick baking dish.
6. Add the chopped spinach, cherry tomatoes, bell peppers, onion, and zucchini evenly on top of eggs.
7. Pour the remaining egg mixture over the vegetables, keeping the space on the top.
8. Make sure that the eggs evenly coat the vegetables.
9. Add the baking dish to the preheated oven.
10. Bake it for 20-25 minutes, or until the omelets are firm and changed to golden on top.
11. Once cooked through, remove the baked vegetable omelets from the oven and allow them to cool slightly before serving.
12. Carefully run a knife around the edges of the omelets to loosen them.
13. Then, gently slide them out onto plates.
14. Garnished with fresh herbs if desired, and serve and enjoy as a hearty breakfast.

Cinnamon Quinoa Porridge

Ingredients:

- 1/2 cup quinoa
- 1 cup almond milk or coconut milk
- 1/2 teaspoon ground cinnamon
- 2 small red apples, diced
- 1/4 cup walnuts, chopped
- 1 tablespoon honey (optional for sweetness)

Nutritional Values per Serving:

Calories   599
% Daily Value*

Total Fat 38.4g   49%

Saturated Fat 26.4g 132%

Cholesterol 0mg   0%

Sodium 22mg   1%

Total Carbohydrate 64g   23%

Dietary Fiber 11g   39%

Total Sugars 36g

Protein 10g

 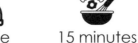

Simple   15 minutes   2

15-20 minutes   30-35 minutes

Directions:

1. The first step is to wash and rinse the quinoa underwater using a fine-mesh sieve.
2. Take a medium saucepan and add the rinsed quinoa and almond milk.
3. Let this mixture come to a boil on medium flame,
4. Once the boil comes, lower the heat and simmer for 15 minutes, covered.
5. Till then, quinoa will absorb all the milk.
6. Add in the ground cinnamon, diced apple, and chopped walnuts.
7. Let it cook for 3-4 minutes.
8. Keep stirring occasionally until the apple is softened and the mixture is heated well.
9. Drizzle the cinnamon quinoa porridge with honey for added sweetness.
10. Serve the porridge warm in bowls as a delicious breakfast after garnishing it with extra cinnamon or a sprinkle of chopped walnuts.

Oatmeal and Blueberry Muffins

Ingredients:

1. 1 cup rolled oats
2. 1 cup fresh blueberries
3. 1/2 cup greek yogurt
4. 2 eggs, whisked
5. 1/4 cup honey
6. ½ teaspoon baking powder

Simple   10 minutes

                         2

18-20 minutes   30 minutes

Nutritional Values per Serving:

Calories   442
% Daily Value*
Total Fat 14g 18%
Saturated Fat 4.1g   20%
Cholesterol 373mg   124%
Sodium 175mg   8%
Total Carbohydrate 64.9g 24%
Dietary Fiber 6.8g   24%
Total Sugars 17.5g
Protein 22.1a

Directions:

1. Before starting the cooking, preheat the oven to 375 degrees F.
2. Then, take a muffin tin and line it with muffin paper.
3. In a large mixing bowl, add blueberries, oats, eggs, honey, Greek yogurt, and baking powder.
4. Whisk all the ingredients well until muffin batter is prepared.
5. Pour this prepared batter into the prepared muffin cups, filling each cup about 1/3 full.
6. Add the muffins to the preheated oven and bake for 18-20 minutes or until they are golden brown.
7. Once the toothpick inserted into the muffin center comes out clean, it's done.
8. Take out the muffins and let them cool in the pan for 10-12 minutes.
9. Next, transfer all to a wire rack and let it cool completely.
10. Serve the oatmeal and blueberry muffins as a delicious and nutritious breakfast or snack option!

Baked Avocado and Egg Toast

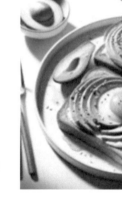

Ingredients:

- 2 slices whole wheat bread
- 1 ripe avocado, peeled, pitted and sliced
- 2 eggs
- 1 tablespoon of sesame seeds

Simple   12 minutes

 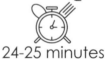
                         2

12-15 minutes   24-25 minutes

Nutritional Values per Serving:

Calories   371
% Daily Value*
Total Fat 27.8g   36%
Saturated Fat 6.2g   31%
Cholesterol 186mg   62%
Sodium 209mg   9%
Total Carbohydrate 21.7g 8%
Dietary Fiber 9.2g   33%
Total Sugars 2.5g
Protein 12.6g

Directions:

1. The first step is to preheat the oven to 370 degrees F.
2. Take a large baking sheet and line it with parchment paper.
3. Take a fresh organic avocado and slice it in half.
4. Put the avocado halves on the prepared baking sheet and cut side up.
5. Slice a small piece off the bottom of each avocado half to create a stable base.
6. Crack one egg into each avocado half.
7. Add the baking sheet inside the oven and bake for 12-15 minutes.
8. Meanwhile, toast the whole wheat bread slices until golden.
9. Once it's cooked, remove it from the oven and let it cool.
10. Transfer one baked avocado half on each slice of toasted whole wheat bread. Season it with sesame seeds.
11. Enjoy this delicious and nutritious breakfast.

Chia and Coconut Pudding

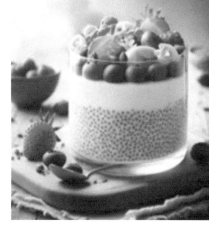

Ingredients:

- 1/4 cup chia seeds
- 1 cup coconut milk
- 1/2 teaspoon vanilla extract
- 1 tablespoon maple syrup (or to taste)
- ¼ cup blueberries
- ½ cup diced strawberries
- 1 banana, sliced

Nutritional Values per Serving:

Calories 529
% Daily Value*
Total Fat 34.5g 44%
Saturated Fat 30.2g 151%
Cholesterol 0mg 0%
Sodium 26mg 1%
Total Carbohydrate 57.5g 21%
Dietary Fiber 5.7g 21%
Total Sugars 43g
Protein 4.1g

Simple — 4 hours 15 minutes — 0 minutes — 24-25 minutes — 2

Directions:

1. In a large mixing bowl, whisk together the coconut milk, chia seeds, vanilla extract, and maple syrup.
2. Mix it well for acceptable incorporation.
3. Pour this mixture evenly between serving glasses or jars.
4. Cover the jars, let them sit inside, and refrigerate them for at least 4 hours or overnight.
5. The time will allow the chia seeds to thicken.
6. Once it's set, remove it from the refrigerator.
7. Stir the pudding and then top with blueberries, sliced bananas, and diced strawberries.

Homemade Energy Bars

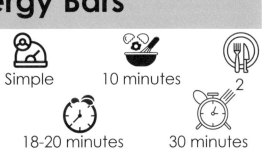

Ingredients:

- 1/2 cup rolled oats
- 1/2 cup pitted dates
- 1/4 cup natural peanut butter
- 2 tablespoons ground flaxseed
- 2 tablespoons chopped walnuts
- 2 tablespoons dark chocolate chips

Simple — 10 minutes — 18-20 minutes — 30 minutes — 2

Nutritional Values per Serving:

Calories 399
% Daily Value*
Total Fat 18.8g 24%
Saturated Fat 4.5g 23%
Cholesterol 0mg 0%
Sodium 7mg 0%
Total Carbohydrate 50.8g 18%
Dietary Fiber 7.7g 28%
Total Sugars 25.1g
Protein 12g

Directions:

1. We are starting the process by preheating your oven to 350 degrees F.
2. Take a small baking dish and line it with parchment paper.
3. Take a high-speed blender and pulse the rolled oats until they have a coarse flour-like texture.
4. Next, add the pitted dates to the food processor.
5. Let it pulse until it form a sticky paste.
6. Transfer this mixture to a mixing bowl.
7. Add the natural peanut butter, ground flaxseed, chopped walnuts, and dark chocolate chips.
8. Mix all the ingredients well until combined.
9. Remember that this mixture should be sticky and hold together when pressed.
10. Line a baking sheet with parchment paper.
11. Transfer this prepared mixture to the baking dish and press it down firmly.
12. Add the baking dish inside the oven and bake it for 18-20 minutes.
13. Serve alongside your morning coffee.
14. Remove the dish from the oven.
15. Let it cool completely.
16. Once cooled, use a sharp knife to cut it into bars.

Berry and Spinach Smoothie

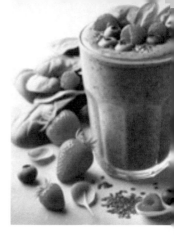

Ingredients:

- ½ cup strawberries
- ½ cup blueberries
- 1/3 cup raspberries
- 1 cup fresh spinach leaves
- 1/2 cup fat-free greek yogurt
- 1/2 cup almond milk
- 1 tablespoon ground flaxseed
- ice cubes for chilling

Nutritional Values per Serving:

Calories   389
% Daily Value*
Total Fat 22.2g   28%
Saturated Fat 7.5g   37%
Cholesterol 1mg   0%
Sodium 80mg   3%
Total Carbohydrate 28.5g   10%
Dietary Fiber 17.4g   62%
Total Sugars 8.5g
Protein 14.4a

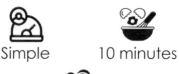

Simple   10 minutes   2

0 minutes   10 minutes

Directions:

1. First, wash and rinse well all the berries.
2. Remove any stems from the berries.
3. In a high-speed blender, combine the mixed berries, spinach leaves, fat-free Greek yogurt, almond milk, and ground flaxseed.
4. Blend it until smooth in consistency.
5. Pour more almond milk until you reach your desired consistency.
6. Top the smoothie with a few extra berries.
7. Enjoy.

Herbed Omelets with Tomatoes and Feta Cheese

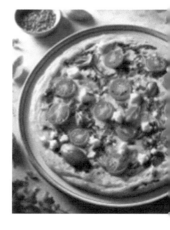

Ingredients:

- 4 eggs
- 2 tablespoons basil finely chopped
- 3 teaspoons of parsley, chopped
- 1/2 cup cherry tomatoes, halved
- 1/4 cup feta cheese, crumbled
- 1/4 cup red onion, finely chopped

Nutritional Values per Serving:

Calories 253
% Daily Value*
Total Fat 19.9g   26%
Saturated Fat 6.6g   33%
Cholesterol 344mg   115%
Sodium 343mg   15%
Total Carbohydrate 5.2g   2%
Dietary Fiber 1.2g 4%
Total Sugars 3.1g   Protein 14.6g

 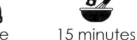

Simple   15 minutes   2

5 minutes   15 minutes

Directions:

1. Take a medium-sized mixing bowl and crack eggs in it.
2. Add in basil and parsley and mix it well.
3. Heat a nonstick skillet over medium heat.
4. Add the egg mixture to the greased skillet, spreading it evenly across the bottom. Let the eggs cook for 1-2 minutes or until the edges start to set.
5. Now, evenly distribute the cherry tomatoes, crumbled feta cheese, and chopped red onion on top of the eggs.
6. Use a spatula to carefully fold the other half of the omelet over the filling to create a half-moon shape.
7. Press down well to seal the omelet.
8. Cook it for 2 minutes or until the omelet is cooked.
9. Serve the omelet onto a plate.
10. Serve and enjoy.

Chapter 6

LUNCH RECIPES

Section 1: White Meat Recipes

Chicken with Lemon and Rosemary

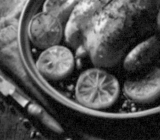

Ingredients:

- 2 chicken breasts, 6 ounces each
- 1 lemon
- 2-3 sprigs of fresh rosemary
- 2 cloves of garlic, minced
- 1 tablespoon chopped fresh basil
- 1 tablespoon chopped fresh parsley

Nutritional Values per Serving:

Calories 167
% Daily Value*
Total Fat 3.2g 4%
Saturated Fat 0.9g 5%
Cholesterol 73mg 24%
Sodium 62mg 3%
Total Carbohydrate 6.4g 2%
Dietary Fiber 2g 7%
Total Sugars 1.3g
Protein28.4g

 Simple 15 minutes 2

 25 minutes 40 minutes

Directions:

1. Preheat your oven to 375 degrees F.
2. Wash and rinse the chicken breasts well under water.
3. Next, pat dry it with a paper towel.
4. Now, take a mixing bowl and add lemon juice and zest, rosemary, garlic, basil, and parsley.
5. Mix it very well.
6. Add chicken breast pieces to it and mix well for a delicate coating.
7. Marinate the chicken for about 1-2 hours in the refrigerator.
8. Take a baking dish and line it with parchment paper.
9. Add the chicken breast pieces to it
10. Add it inside the oven and bake it for 25-30 minutes.
11. Once cooked, please remove the baking dish from the oven and let it rest for a few minutes.
12. Serve the lemon rosemary chicken breasts hot.
13. Enjoy.

Turkey Stuffed with Spinach

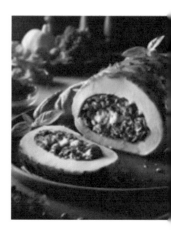

Ingredients:

- 2 pounds of turkey breast
- 2 cups fresh spinach, chopped
- 1/2 cup low-fat ricotta cheese
- 1/4 teaspoon nutmeg
- 2 tablespoons fresh basil, chopped
- 2 tablespoons fresh parsley, chopped

Nutritional Values per Serving:

Calories 116
% Daily Value*
Total Fat 3.8g 5%
Saturated Fat 1.5g 8%
Cholesterol 42mg 14%
Sodium 91mg 4%
Total Carbohydrate 2.7g 1%
Dietary Fiber 1.2g 4%
Total Sugars 0.3g
Protein 17.6g

 Simple 15 minutes 4

 60 minutes 75 minutes

Directions:

1. Preheat the oven to 375 degrees F.
2. Wash the turkey breast under water and pat dry with a paper towel.
3. Take a knife and butterfly the turkey breast by slicing it horizontally along the side.
4. It will create a pocket for stuffing
5. Now; start preparing the stuffing; for that, take a bowl and combine the chopped spinach, low-fat ricotta cheese, nutmeg, chopped basil, and chopped parsley, and mix it well.
6. Stuff the Turkey Breast with the prepared mixture.
7. Next, fold the turkey breast back together to enclose the stuffing.
8. Seal the edges as well.
9. Add the stuffed turkey breast in a roasting pan lined with parchment paper.
10. Cook it for 60-70 minutes until the turkey's internal temperature reaches 165 degrees F.
11. Remove turkey breasts from the oven
12. And let them rest for about 15 minutes before slicing.
13. Enjoy afterward.

Grilled Chicken with Avocado Sauce

Ingredients:

- 2 chicken breasts, 6 ounces each
- 2 large ripe avocados
- 2 tablespoons of lime juice
- ½ cup of fresh coriander, chopped
- 8 cherry tomatoes, halved

Nutritional Values per Serving:

Calories   491
% Daily Value*
Total Fat 27.8g   36%
Saturated Fat 6.3g   31%
Cholesterol 89mg   30%
Sodium 114mg   5%
Total Carbohydrate 32.6g   12%
Dietary Fiber 12g   43%
Total Sugars 12.7g
Protein 34.8g

Simple   15 minutes   2
25 minutes   35 minutes

Directions:

1. The first step is to preheat the grill at medium to high heat.
2. Next, rinse the chicken breasts under cold water.
3. Then pat dry it with paper towels.
4. Coat the grilled skillet with oil spray, and add breast to it
5. , and grill for 6 minutes per side.
6. Meanwhile, prepare avocado sauce.
7. Remove the pit of avocados and scoop out the flesh.
8. Add it to a food processor.
9. Add the lime juice, cherry tomatoes, and add chopped coriander.
10. Blend until smooth and creamy. Serve it with grilled chicken.
11. Enjoy.

Chicken Strips with Peppers

Ingredients:

- 1.5 pounds of chicken breast, cut into strips
- 2 bell peppers (mix color), sliced
- 1 onion, sliced
- 2 teaspoons paprika
- 1 teaspoon dried thyme

Nutritional Values per Serving:

Calories   144
% Daily Value*
Total Fat 2.2g 3%
Saturated Fat 0g   0%
Cholesterol 48mg   16%
Sodium 43mg   2%
Total Carbohydrate 13.7g   5%
Dietary Fiber 2.7g   10%
Total Sugars 8.1g
Protein 17.7g

Simple   12 minutes   2
12 minutes   24 minutes

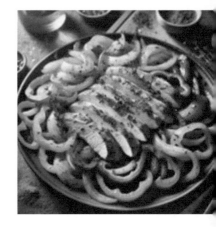

Directions:

1. Preheat the grill for a few minutes before starting the cooking process.
2. Next, prepare the chicken strips by tossing them with bell pepper, onions, paprika, and thyme.
3. Thread chicken strips onto wooden skewers alternating between the veggies.
4. Mist the grill grate with oil spray.
5. Grill the skewers for 8-12 minutes, turning them occasionally until appropriately cooked.
6. Serve hot, and enjoy.

Baked Turkey and Pumpkin

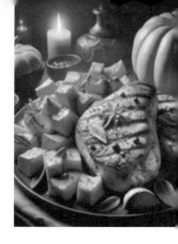

Ingredients:

- 2 pounds of turkey breast
- 1 pumpkin, peeled, seedless, and chunked
- 6 fresh sage leaves, chopped
- 6 cloves of garlic, minced
- Handful of fresh parsley, chopped

Nutritional Values per Serving:

Calories   115
% Daily Value*
Total Fat 4.1g 5%
Saturated Fat 1.3g   6%
Cholesterol 33mg   11%
Sodium 34mg   1%
Total Carbohydrate 8.3g   3%
Dietary Fiber 3.1g   11%
Total Sugars 2.1g
Protein 12.2g

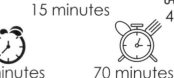

Simple   15 minutes   4

55 minutes   70 minutes

Directions:

1. Before starting the cooking, let's preheat the oven to 375 degrees F.
2. Rinse the turkey breasts under runny water and pat it dry with paper towels.
3. Add the turkey breasts in a roasting pan lined with parchment paper.
4. Add the chunked pumpkin pieces beside the turkey breasts.
5. Season the turkey and pumpkin with chopped sage leaves and minced garlic.
6. Cover this baking dish with aluminum foil.
7. Then, add it to the oven.
8. Bake for about 45-55 minutes.
9. Once tender, remove the baking dish from the oven, and let it rest for 15 minutes.
10. Cut the turkey breasts into slices and serve them with the baked pumpkin.
11. Garnish with fresh parsley and enjoy.

Light Chicken Curry

Ingredients:

- 1 pound of chicken breasts, diced
- 12 ounces of light coconut milk
- 2 tablespoons curry powder
- 1 large zucchini, sliced
- Handful of fresh coriander, chopped

Nutritional Values per Serving:

Calories   72
% Daily Value*
Total Fat 1.4g 2%
Saturated Fat 0.1g   1%
Cholesterol 0mg   0%
Sodium 6mg 0%
Total Carbohydrate 2.9g   1%
Dietary Fiber 1.2g   4%
Total Sugars 0.9g
Protein 13.4g

Simple   15 minutes   2

25 minutes   40 minutes

Directions:

1. First, rinse the chicken breast and pat dry with a paper towel.
2. Take a large cooking pot that is non–stick and heat it over medium flame.
3. Then add to it diced chicken breasts.
4. Just cook it enough that it changes color.
5. Next, add the sliced zucchini to the pot and continue cooking until the zucchini is slightly tender.
6. Pour in the Coconut Milk and remaining listed ingredients.
7. Pour the light coconut milk into the pot with the chicken and zucchini.
8. Mix and simmer it for 15 minutes, covered.
9. Adjust curry seasoning and serve it with a garnish of coriander.

Mediterranean Chicken Salad

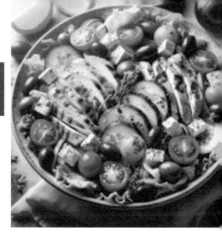

Ingredients:

- 2 grilled chicken breasts, sliced
- 4 cups lettuce, chopped (romaine or mixed greens)
- 1 cup cherry tomatoes, halved
- 1 cucumber, sliced
- 1/2 cup pitted Kalamata olives
- 1/2 cup low-fat feta cheese, crumbled
- 1 lemon, cut into wedges
- 1 teaspoon dried oregano

Simple   15 minutes   3

12 minutes   27 minutes

Nutritional Values per Serving:

Calories   140
% Daily Value*
Total Fat 4.4g   6%
Saturated Fat 0.6g   3%
Cholesterol 44mg   15%
Sodium 247mg 11%
Total Carbohydrate 9.9g   4%
Dietary Fiber 2.7g   10%
Total Sugars 3.3g
Protein 16.5g

Directions:

1. The first step is to preheat the grill for a few minutes and mist the grill grate with oil spray.
2. Cook the chicken breasts for 6 minutes per side at medium heat.
3. Meanwhile, prepare the salad by combining lettuce, cherry tomatoes, cucumber, olives, and feta cheese.
4. Pour the lemon juice on top and then season it with dried oregano.
5. Toss the salad well.
6. Dice the grilled and cooked chicken breast pieces and then top it over the salad.
7. Serve and enjoy.

Grilled Chicken Breast with Mixed Vegetables

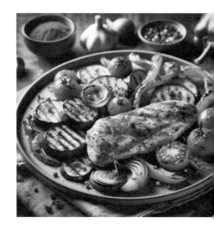

Ingredients:

- 2 skinless chicken breasts
- 2 medium zucchinis, sliced
- 1 red pepper, sliced
- 1 red onion, sliced
- 1 cup cherry tomatoes
- 1 teaspoon garlic powder
- 1 teaspoon sweet paprika
- 1 teaspoon dried oregano

Simple   15 minutes   2

12 minutes   27 minutes

Nutritional Values per Serving:

Calories   259
% Daily Value*
Total Fat 7.9g 10%
Saturated Fat 2.1g   10%
Cholesterol 89mg   30%
Sodium 102mg   4%
Total Carbohydrate 15.5g   6%
Dietary Fiber 3.7g   13%
Total Sugars 8.5g
Protein 32g

Directions:

1. The first step is to preheat the grill to medium level.
2. Next, rub the chicken breasts with garlic powder, sweet paprika, and dried oregano on both sides.
3. Take a medium-sized mixing bowl and add red peppers, sliced zucchini, red onions, and cherry tomatoes, and toss all these ingredients well.
4. Add the seasoned chicken breasts to the preheated grill.
5. Grill the chicken for about 6 minutes each side.
6. Meanwhile, add the mixed vegetables on a piece of foil over the grill grates beside the chicken.
7. Grill it for 10 minutes, tossing occasionally
8. Once the chicken and vegetables are tender, remove them from the grill.
9. Serve the grilled chicken breasts with mixed vegetables.
10. Enjoy!

SECTION 2:

Vegetarian Recipes

Vegetarian Chili

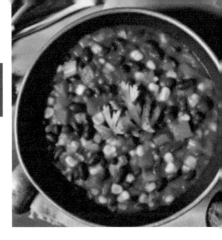

Ingredients:

- 14 ounces of canned black beans, rinsed and drained
- 2 cups corn kernels (fresh, frozen, or canned)
- 1 bell pepper, diced
- 14 ounces of diced tomatoes
- 1 onion, diced
- 2 teaspoons ground cumin
- 2 teaspoons ground coriander

Nutritional Values per Serving:

Calories   432
% Daily Value*
Total Fat 2.6g 3%
Saturated Fat 0.5g   3%
Cholesterol 0mg   0%
Sodium 22mg   1%
Total Carbohydrate 83.1g   30%
Dietary Fiber 18.9g   67%
Total Sugars 9.5g
Protein 24.8g

Simple   10 minutes   4

30 minutes   40 minutes

Directions:

1. Take a large Dutch oven and heat it over medium flame.
2. Add a splash of water to it to prevent sticking.
3. Now put the diced onion and bell pepper in the Dutch oven and cook for 5 minutes, stirring frequently.
4. Next, add the black beans, diced tomatoes (with juices), and corn kernels.
5. Add the ground cumin and ground coriander for seasoning.
6. Stir it well.
7. Let this chili simmer and lower the heat.
8. Cover the Dutch oven and cook the chili for 20 minutes
9. Adjust the seasoning if needed, adding cumin.
10. Serve the vegetarian chili hot.
11. Enjoy.

Quinoa and Roasted Vegetables

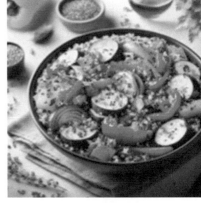

Ingredients:

- 1 cup quinoa
- 1 zucchini, diced
- 1 bell pepper (any color), diced
- 1 red onion, diced
- 2 carrots, diced
- 1 teaspoon dried thyme
- 2 tablespoons fresh parsley, chopped

Nutritional Values per Serving:

Calories   406
% Daily Value*
Total Fat 5.6g 7%
Saturated Fat 0.6g   3%
Cholesterol 0mg   0%
Sodium 88mg   4%
Total Carbohydrate 76.2g   28%
Dietary Fiber 11.4g   41%
Total Sugars 11g
Protein 14.9g

Simple   25 minutes   2

40 minutes   65 minutes

Directions:

1. First, wash and rinse the quinoa under tap water to remove all the bitterness; use a fine-mesh sieve for this.
2. Take a saucepan and add the rinsed quinoa and water.
3. Cook the quinoa until the boil comes.
4. Then, reduce the heat to low and cook with a cover on top for 15 minutes.
5. Till then, the quinoa will absorb all the liquids.
6. Mix and fluff the quinoa with a fork and set it aside for further use.
7. Now, preheat your oven to 375 degrees F.
8. Add the diced zucchini, bell pepper, red onion, and carrots in a large mixing bowl.
9. Toss veggies well and season with dried thyme and toss again to coat the veggies.
10. Layer the seasoned vegetables on a baking sheet lined with parchment paper.
11. Roast it inside the oven for about 20-25 minutes
12. Now transfer veggies to a large bowl and add cooked quinoa.
13. Toss well and then serve with garnish of parsley.

Greek Salad with Chickpeas

Ingredients:

- 14 ounces of chickpeas, drained and rinsed
- 2 large tomatoes, diced
- 2 small cucumber, diced
- 1/3 cup pitted kalamata olives
- 6 ounces of low-fat feta cheese, crumbled
- 1 teaspoon dried oregano
- juice of 1 lemon

Nutritional Values per Serving:

Calories   404
% Daily Value*
Total Fat 7.9g   10%
Saturated Fat 1.3g   6%
Cholesterol 3mg   1%
Sodium 185mg8%
Total Carbohydrate 65.4g   24%
Dietary Fiber 18.7g   67%
Total Sugars 12.9g
Protein 21.4g

Simple   15 minutes   4

0 minutes   15 minutes

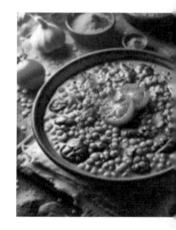

Directions:

1. Start the cooking by draining and rinsing the chickpeas thoroughly under cold water.
2. This helps remove excess sodium and any canning liquid. Set aside.
3. Once vegetables are diced and prepared, add them to a mixing bowl along with rinsed chickpeas.
4. Season it with dried oregano and toss the salad to coat it evenly.
5. Squeeze the juice of one lemon over the salad.
6. Gently toss again and serve it once combined by adding feta cheese on top.

Red Lentil Curry

Ingredients:

- 1 cup red lentils
- 14 ounces of light coconut milk
- 2 tablespoons curry powder
- 2 cups fresh spinach leaves, chopped
- 2 red large tomatoes, diced
- 1 cup of fresh coriander leaves for garnish

Nutritional Values per Serving:

Calories   455
% Daily Value*
Total Fat 31.4g   40%
Saturated Fat 26.2g 131%
Cholesterol 5mg   2%
Sodium 266mg   12%
Total Carbohydrate 36g   13%
Dietary Fiber 12.9g   46%
Total Sugars 7g
Protein 14.3g

Simple   20 minutes   4

30-40 minutes   50 minutes

Directions:

1. The first step is to remove debris and excess dirt from the lentils and rinse under cold water until the water runs clear.
2. Combine the rinsed red lentils with the light coconut milk in a large saucepan.
3. Stir in the curry powder and let it cook until the boil comes.
4. Lower the flame and let it cook for 10 minutes.
5. Next, cover and cook for 10 more minutes.
6. Afterward, add spinach and tomatoes, and cook in simmering mode for 10 minutes.
7. Before serving the dish, garnish the Red Lentil Curry with fresh coriander leaves.
8. Enjoy.

Black Bean Tacos

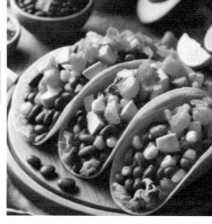

Ingredients:

- 8 ounces of black beans, drained and rinsed
- 1-1/4 cup corn kernels (fresh, frozen, or canned)
- 1 cup shredded lettuce
- 2 tomatoes, diced
- 1 avocado, diced
- fresh coriander leaves for garnish
- lime wedges for serving

Nutritional Values per Serving:

Calories 377
% Daily Value*
Total Fat 21.7g 28%
Saturated Fat 4.3g   22%
Cholesterol 0mg   0%
Sodium 54mg 2%
Total Carbohydrate 45.1g   16%
Dietary Fiber 16.7g   59%
Total Sugars 7.9g
Protein 10.4g

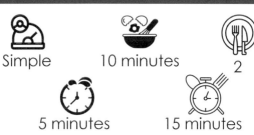

Simple   10 minutes   2

5 minutes   15 minutes

Directions:

1. Drained and rinsed the black beans.
2. Take a medium saucepan and heat the black beans over medium flame until warm.
3. Then add the corn kernels to it and stir to combine.
4. Let it cook for another 3-5 minutes,
5. Layer shredded lettuce leaves onto a flat plate.
6. Divide the black bean and corn mixture on top of lettuce leaves equally.
7. Top it with diced avocado, diced tomatoes,
8. Sprinkle fresh coriander leaves over the lettuce tacos.
9. Serve the tacos with lime wedges.

Crispy Quinoa and Veggie Wrap

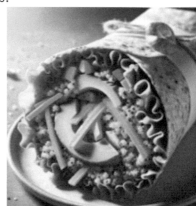

Ingredients:

- 1/2 cup cooked quinoa
- 2 lettuce leaves
- 1/2 carrot, julienned
- 1/4 bell pepper (color of choice), sliced
- 1/4 avocado, sliced
- 1 whole wheat tortilla

Nutritional Values per Serving:

Calories: Approx. 350
Total Fat: 9g (12%)
Saturated Fat: 1.5g (8%)
Cholesterol: 0mg (0%)
Sodium: 200mg (9%)
Total Carbohydrates: 58g (21%)
Dietary Fiber: 9g (32%)
Total Sugars: 3g
Protein: 9g

Easy   10 minutes   1

0 minutes   10 minutes

Directions:

1. Wash the lettuce, peel and julienne the carrot, slice the bell pepper, and slice the avocado.
2. Lay the whole wheat tortilla on a plate or cutting board.
3. Place the lettuce leaves in the center of the tortilla as a base for the other ingredients. This helps keep the wrap compact and prevents moist ingredients from making the tortilla too soft.
4. Add the cooked quinoa over the lettuce, spreading it evenly.
5. Carefully arrange the carrot strips, bell pepper slices, and avocado slices on top of the quinoa.
6. Carefully fold the tortilla, folding the sides towards the center and then rolling it up tightly from the side nearest to you towards the opposite side, to close the wrap.
7. If desired, the wrap can be cut in half for easier eating.

Barley and Vegetable Soup

Ingredients:

- 1.5 cups barley
- 2 large carrots, diced
- 2 stalks of celery, diced
- 4 tomatoes, diced
- 2 cups fresh spinach leaves, chopped
- 1 teaspoon dried rosemary
- 4 cloves garlic, minced
- 1/4 cup fresh parsley, chopped

Nutritional Values per Serving:

Calories   386
% Daily Value*
Total Fat 2.8g 4%
Saturated Fat 0.5g   3%
Cholesterol 0mg   0%
Sodium 254mg   11%
Total Carbohydrate 80.1g   29%
Dietary Fiber 22.1g   79%
Total Sugars 12.7g
Protein 15.9g

Simple   20 minutes   2

1 hour 10 minutes   1 hour 30 minutes

Directions:

1. The first step is to prepare the barley well underwater using a fine-mesh sieve.
2. Then, remove all the debris and set it aside.
3. Take a nonstick skillet or pot and add minced garlic with a splash of water or cook.
4. Let it cook for 1 minute. Add diced carrots and celery to the pot and cook for 5 minutes. Add the rinsed barley, tomatoes, spinach, and rosemary.
5. Let it cook for 3 minutes.
6. Then, add enough water to ensure the barley gets cooked and the ingredients are submerged.
7. Let this soup boil, then reduce the heat to low
8. Covered it and simmer for 1 hour.
9. Stir in the chopped parsley for a final burst of freshness.
10. Serve and enjoy it hot.

Whole Wheat Pasta Primavera

Ingredients:

- 10 ounces of whole-wheat pasta
- 1 cup of trimmed fresh asparagus, cut into small pieces
- 1 -1/4 cup peeled peas, fresh
- 1 cup carrots, thinly sliced
- 1 large zucchini, diced
- 4 tablespoons extra virgin olive oil
- 4 cloves garlic, minced
- juice of 1 lemon
- ½ cup of parmesan cheese, grated and for serving

Nutritional Values per Serving:

Calories   571
% Daily Value*
Total Fat 18.2g   23%
Saturated Fat 6.7g   33%
Cholesterol 27mg   9%
Sodium 1060mg   46%
Total Carbohydrate 83.4g   30%
Dietary Fiber 9g   32%
Total Sugars 11.1g
Protein 21.6g

Simple   20 minutes   6

30 minutes   50 minutes

Directions:

1. The first step is to cook the whole wheat pasta according to the package instructions.
2. Then drain and set it aside.
3. Add olive oil to the skillet.
4. Then sauté the garlic until the aroma comes over medium flame.
5. Then add carrots and diced zucchini and cook for 3-4 minutes until they soften.
6. Next, mix the asparagus pieces and peas into the skillet and cook for 3-4 minutes until the vegetables are tender.
7. Next, add cooked pasta to veggies skillet
8. Pasta and Vegetables:
9. Add lemon juice over the pasta and vegetables, tossing gently to combine.
10. Top the grated Parmesan cheese over the top of each serving.
11. Serve and enjoy.

Tomato and Basil Risotto

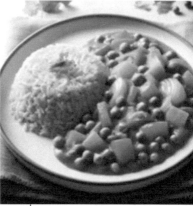

Ingredients:

- 1 cup arborio rice
- 16 ounces of peeled tomatoes, diced
- 6 cups low-sodium vegetable broth
- 1 cup fresh basil leaves, chopped
- 4 cloves garlic, minced
- 2 tablespoons olive oil

Simple   15 minutes   2

30 minutes   45 minutes

Nutritional Values per Serving:

Calories	350	
% Daily Value*		
Total Fat 14.6g		19%
Saturated Fat 2.1g		10%
Cholesterol 0mg		0%
Sodium 283mg		12%
Total Carbohydrate 46.4g		17%
Dietary Fiber 3.2g		11%
Total Sugars 1.1g		
Protein 7.5g		

Directions:

1. Take a large cooking pot and pour vegetable broth in it.
2. Simmer it at low and keep it cooking process.
3. Heat the vegetable broth over low heat, keeping it warm throughout the cooking process.
4. Take a Dutch oven and heat the olive oil.
5. Add the Arborio rice to cook the minced garlic until the aroma comes.
6. Cook the rice for 1-2 minutes until it becomes translucent around the edges.
7. Add the diced tomatoes into the saucepan, stirring occasionally.
8. Now, pour warm vegetable broth into the rice mixture and let it cook until it is creamy.
9. It should take about 18-20 minutes.
10. Add the basil leaves once the risotto is cooked, reserving a few for garnish.
11. Serve it immediately.

Brown Rice with Vegetable Curry

Ingredients:

- 1 cup brown rice
- 12 ounces of low-fat coconut milk
- 2 tablespoons curry powder
- 1 large white onion, diced
- 1 bell pepper, diced
- 1 cup peas, fresh
- ½ cup of coriander leaves for garnish
- 2 small carrots, diced

Simple   20 minutes   4

 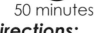 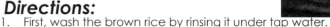

50 minutes   70 minutes

Nutritional Values per Serving:

Calories	433	
% Daily Value*		
Total Fat 29.7g		38%
Saturated Fat 25.5g		128%
Cholesterol 0mg		0%
Sodium 63mg		3%
Total Carbohydrate 39.9g		14%
Dietary Fiber 7.6g		27%
Total Sugars 10.6g		
Protein 7.4g		

Directions:

1. First, wash the brown rice by rinsing it under tap water.
2. Remove all the excess starch under water and run clean.
3. Take a nonstick saucepan and add the rice to it with 2 cups of water.
4. Let the water boil, then reduce the heat to low, cover, and simmer for 45-50 minutes.
5. Meanwhile, take a large skillet and add coconut milk to a small amount. Heat it over medium flame, and then add diced onion to the skillet and sauté for 5 minutes until translucent.
6. Stir in the diced carrots and bell pepper, and cook for 5 minutes until the vegetables soften.
7. Now, pour the remaining coconut milk into it as well.
8. Fluff the cooked rice with a fork.
9. Add the curry powder, ensuring the veggies are sautéed well.
10. Next, put the peas into the skillet and cook for 15 minutes.
11. Once the rice and veggies are cooked, serve them by fluffing them with a fork on a serving plate and topping them with the cooked veggies.
12. Enjoy the dish hot.

Whole meal Spaghetti with Avocado Pesto

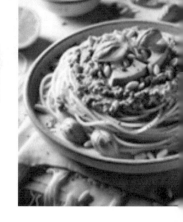

Ingredients:

- 12 ounces of whole-wheat spaghetti
- 2 ripe avocado, pitted and skin removed
- 1 cup fresh basil leaves
- ½ cup pine nuts
- 4 cloves garlic, minced
- Juice of 1 lemon
- 2 -4 tablespoons extra virgin olive oil

 Simple 15 minutes 4

 20 minutes 35 minutes

Nutritional Values per Serving:

Calories   339
% Daily Value*
Total Fat 25.8g 33%
Saturated Fat 3.7g   19%
Cholesterol 0mg   0%
Sodium 6mg   0%
Total Carbohydrate 25.2g   9%
Dietary Fiber 7.4g   26%
Total Sugars 1.3g
Protein 7.2g

Directions:

1. First, cook the whole wheat spaghetti pasta according to package instructions until al dente.
2. Then drain and set aside, reserving a small amount of pasta water for further use.
3. Take a high-speed blender and pulse together the flesh of the ripe avocado, fresh basil leaves, pine nuts, minced garlic, and lemon juice.
4. Pulse it until well blended.
5. Slowly add extra virgin olive oil to prepare pesto when it's blending.
6. Toss the cooked whole wheat spaghetti with the prepared avocado pesto in a large mixing bowl until the pasta is evenly coated.
7. If the pesto is too thick, you can add a splash of reserved pasta water
8. Serve and enjoy.

Baked Salmon with Herbs

Ingredients:

- 2 salmon fillets (about 6 ounces each)
- 2 lemon, thinly sliced
- ½ cup of fresh dill sprigs
- ½ cup of fresh parsley, chopped
- 4 cloves garlic, minced

 Simple 15 minutes 2

 12-15 minutes 30 minutes

Nutritional Values per Serving:

Calories   180
% Daily Value*
Total Fat 6.7g 9%
Saturated Fat 1g   5%
Cholesterol 44mg   15%
Sodium 62mg   3%
Total Carbohydrate 13g   5%
Dietary Fiber 3.8g   14%
Total Sugars 2.8g
Protein 21.7g

Directions:

1. Pat dries the salmon fillet with a paper towel.
2. Take a pestle and mortar and add garlic, parsley, and dill springs to it
3. Grate it well manually and add 2 lemons juiced to it
4. Make a paste and cover the salmon fillet with it.
5. Next, preheat your oven to 390 degrees F.
6. Then, line a large-sized baking sheet with parchment paper
7. Add salmon to the baking pan.
8. Put the baking sheet into the oven.
9. then bake for 12 minutes, until the salmon is done
10. Then, remove it from the oven and rest for a few minutes.
11. Serve the Oven-Baked Salmon, and enjoy!

Cod Steaks with Pesto

Ingredients:

- 6 cod steaks (about 6 ounces each)
- 1 cup basil pesto
- 2 cups cherry tomatoes, halved
- 1 cup basil leaves for garnish

Nutritional Values per Serving:

Calories   492
% Daily Value*
Total Fat 5.5g 7%
Saturated Fat 0g   0%
Cholesterol 295mg   98%
Sodium 377mg   16%
Total Carbohydrate 1.7g   1%
Dietary Fiber 0.7g   2%
Total Sugars 0.9g
Protein 108g

Simple   10 minutes   6
20 minutes   30 minutes

Directions:

1. First, preheat your oven to 390 degrees F.
2. Then, pat the fish fillet dry with a paper towel.
3. Now coat the fillet with basil pesto.
4. Add it to a baking sheet lined with parchment paper.
5. Put the halved cherry tomatoes beside the cod steaks.
6. Add it inside the oven and bake it for 20 minutes, until the fish gets flaky.
7. Ext. Remove the cod steaks from the oven and let them rest for 5 minutes.
8. Garnish with fresh basil leaves and serve.

Grilled Sea Bream with Quinoa Salad

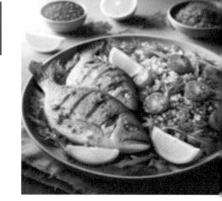

Ingredients:

- Ingredients for Grilled Sea Bream:
- 4 sea bream fillets
- 2 lemons, juice
- 1/4 cup fresh parsley, chopped
- 2 tablespoons fresh dill, chopped
- For Quinoa Salad:
- 1 cup quinoa, cooked
- 2 cups arugula
- 1 cup cherry tomatoes, halved
- 1/4 cup fresh parsley, chopped
- 2 tablespoons fresh dill, chopped
- Juice of 1 lemon

Nutritional Values per Serving:

% Daily Value*
Total Fat 13.2g   17%
Saturated Fat 2.8g   14%
Cholesterol 31mg   10%
Sodium 505mg   22%
Total Carbohydrate 37.7g   14%
Dietary Fiber 4.4g   16%
Total Sugars 2.5g
Protein 19g

Simple   20 minutes   4
15 minutes   35 minutes

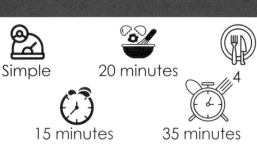

Directions:

1. Preheat the grill to medium flame.
2. Take a food process and add lemon juice, parsley, and dill.
3. Pulse to make a paste
4. Coat the fillet with it and grill for 15 minutes, flipping half way through.
5. Be careful not to overcook.
6. While the sea bream is grilling, add the cooked quinoa, arugula, tomatoes, parsley, and dill to a bowl.
7. Pour the lemon juice over the salad.
8. Then, toss it well.
9. Drop the cooked quinoa with a fork,
10. And divide this salad among plates.
11. Then, top each portion with a grilled sea bream fillet.
12. Garnish with additional lemon, and enjoy.

Sea Bass in Foil with Vegetables

Ingredients:
- 2 sea bass fillets
- 1 zucchini, sliced
- 1 red bell pepper, sliced
- 1 yellow bell pepper, sliced
- 1 cup cherry tomatoes, halved
- fresh thyme sprigs
- 2 cloves garlic, minced

Nutritional Values per Serving:
Calories   164
% Daily Value*
Total Fat 2.9g 4%
Saturated Fat 0.7g   3%
Cholesterol 53mg   18%
Sodium 96mg   4%
Total Carbohydrate 9.1g   3%
Dietary Fiber 2g   7%
Total Sugars 5.2g
Protein 25.5g

Simple   10 minutes

15 minutes   25 minutes

Directions:
1. Preheat the oven to 400 degrees F.
2. Take two large pieces of aluminum foil.
3. Put the sea bass fillet on each piece of foil.
4. Add the thyme leaves, zucchini, tomatoes, bell peppers, and garlic to a large mixing bowl.
5. Toss all the ingredients well.
6. Now, distribute this prepared vegetable mixture equally between the two sea bass fillets, arranging them on top.
7. Fold the foil over the sea bass and vegetables and seal them into packets.
8. Add the foil packets on a baking sheet.
9. Bake it inside the oven for 15 minutes.
10. Once done, transfer the sea bass and vegetables onto serving plates.
11. Serve.

Trout Fillets with Yogurt Sauce

Ingredients:
- 4 trout fillets, 6 ounces each
- 1 cup low-fat greek yogurt
- 1 cucumber, grated
- 2 tablespoons fresh dill, chopped
- 4 cloves of garlic, minced

Nutritional Values per Serving:
Calories   224
% Daily Value*
Total Fat 8.8g 11%
Saturated Fat 1.7g   8%
Cholesterol 75mg   25%
Sodium 82mg   4%
Total Carbohydrate 6.8g   2%
Dietary Fiber 0.3g   1%
Total Sugars 5.1g
Protein 28.1g

Simple   10 minutes

15 minutes   25 minutes

Directions:
1. Preheat your oven to 375 degrees F.
2. Add the parchment paper onto a baking sheet or dish.
3. Add the trout fillets on a baking sheet.
4. Bake the trout fillets in the preheated oven for 12-15 minutes.
5. Meanwhile, in a large mixing bowl, prepare the yogurt sauce by combining the low-fat Greek yogurt, grated cucumber, chopped dill, minced garlic,
6. Mix it well to combine.
7. Once the trout fillets are flaky and cooked, remove it from the oven.
8. Next, let it cool slightly.
9. Serve the trout fillets hot, topped with a generous spoonful of the yogurt sauce.
10. Garnish with additional fresh dill, and enjoy.

Steamed Sea Bass with Ginger

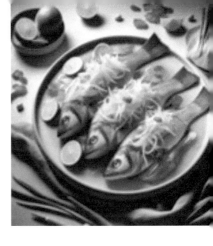

Ingredients:

- 2 sea bass fillets
- 1-inch piece of ginger, julienned
- 2 spring onions, thinly sliced
- Handful of fresh coriander leaves
- 1 lime, sliced

Nutritional Values per Serving:

Calories 171
% Daily Value*
Total Fat 2.9g 4%
Saturated Fat 0.7g 4%
Cholesterol 53mg 18%
Sodium 104mg 5%
Total Carbohydrate 12.6g 5%
Dietary Fiber 4g 14%
Total Sugars 3.2g
Protein 25.8g

Simple 10 minutes 2
10 minutes 20 minutes

Directions:

1. Take a steamer, fill the pot with water, and let it simmer.
2. Season the sea bass fillets with ginger and add it to heat proffer dish.
3. Top the fish with sliced spring.
4. Arrange a few slices of lime on top of the sea bass.
5. Add the heatproof dish to the steamer, cover, and steam for 8-10 minutes,
6. Once cooked, turn off the flame and remove the dish from the steamer.
7. Garnish the steamed sea bass with fresh coriander leaves.
8. Serve hot

Prawn Curry with Coconut Milk

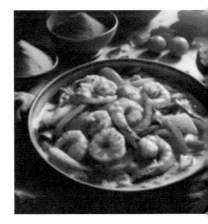

Ingredients:

- 1.5 pounds of prawns, peeled and deveined
- 14 ounces of light coconut milk
- 2 tablespoons curry powder
- 1 -2 red bell pepper, sliced
- 1 yellow bell pepper, sliced
- ½ cup fresh coriander leaves, chopped

Nutritional Values per Serving:

Calories 647
% Daily Value*
Total Fat 58.6g 75%
Saturated Fat 51.1g 256%
Cholesterol 158mg 53%
Sodium 231mg 10%
Total Carbohydrate 15.4g 6%
Dietary Fiber 6g 21%
Total Sugars 8.2g
Protein 23.1g

Simple 10 minutes 2
15 minutes 25 minutes

Directions:

1. Take a nonstick skillet and add a splash of water to it.
2. Next, sprinkle the curry powder and stir for about ½ minute until fragrant.
3. Next, put in the sliced bell peppers and let it cook for 2-3 minutes.
4. Pour in the light coconut milk and bring this mixture to a simmer.
5. Add the prawns to a milk mixture at this stage and cook for 5-7 minutes until they turn pink.
6. Once the prawns are cooked through, remove the skillet from heat.
7. Serve with the topping of chopped coriander leaves over the curry.
8. Serve hot and enjoy.

CHAPTER 7:

DINNER RECIPES

Section 1: Vegetarian Recipes

Eggplant Casserole

Ingredients:

- 2 large eggplants, sliced into 1/4-inch rounds
- 2 cups tomato sauce (homemade or store-bought)
- 1 cup firm tofu, crumbled
- 1/2 cup fresh basil leaves, torn
- 1/4 cup grated parmesan cheese

Nutritional Values per Serving:

Calories   130
% Daily Value*
Total Fat 5.3g   7%
Saturated Fat 2.3g   11%
Cholesterol 9mg   3%
Sodium 649mg28%
Total Carbohydrate 13.2g   5%
Dietary Fiber 5.9g   21%
Total Sugars 7.6g
Protein 11.2g

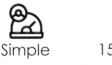 Simple
  15 minutes
 2
35 minutes   50 minutes

Directions:

1. First, before starting the cooking process preheat your oven to 375 degrees F.
2. Prepare the eggplants by heating it in a skillet over medium flame and cooking the slices until golden on both sides.
3. Cook the eggplants in batches.
4. Then, transfer the fried eggplant slices to a large plate.
5. Now it's time to layer the casserole
6. Take a large casserole dish and layer tomato sauce onto the bottom.
7. Now, layer the sauce with fried eggplant slices on top.
8. Sprinkle some crumbled tofu over the eggplant, followed by torn basil leaves.
9. Drizzle a little more tomato sauce over the basil.
10. Repeat these same layering processes until the ingredients are done, finishing with a layer of tomato sauce on top.
11. Top it with shredded parmesan cheese evenly over the top of the casserole.
12. Bake by covering the baking dish with aluminum foil and adding it to the oven for 30 minutes or until the cheese is melted.
13. Once baked, remove the foil and let the casserole cool for a few minutes before serving. Garnish with fresh basil leaves.
14. Enjoy hot.

Lentil and Vegetable Soup

Ingredients:

- 1 cup dried lentils, rinsed and picked over
- 2 carrots, diced
- 2 celery stalks, diced
- 1 cans (14 ounces) diced tomatoes, un-drained
- 6 cups water
- 2 cups fresh spinach leaves, chopped
- 6 cloves garlic, minced

Nutritional Values per Serving:

Calories   139
% Daily Value*
Total Fat 0.6g 1%
Saturated Fat 0.1g   1%
Cholesterol 0mg   0%
Sodium 122mg 5%
Total Carbohydrate 25.7g   9%
Dietary Fiber 11.2g   40%
Total Sugars 4.6g
Protein 9.2g

 Simple
  15 minutes
 4
35 minutes   50 minutes

Directions:

1. First, wash the lentils and pick out all the debris.
2. Then, set it aside for further use.
3. Take a large skillet and add a splash of water to it.
4. Cook the minced garlic for another minute until fragrant.
5. Stir in the diced carrots and celery.
6. Let the vegetables simmer for about 5 minutes, stirring occasionally, until the vegetables get tender.
7. Please put in the diced tomatoes (with their juices) and water. Stir in the rinsed lentils,
8. Let the soup boil, and then reduce the heat to low. Let it simmer for about 25 minutes or until the lentils are tender.
9. Once the lentils are soft, add the chopped spinach leaves. Let it simmer again for 5 minutes or until the spinach is wilted.
10. Ladle the hot lentil and vegetable soup into bowls.
11. Garnish each of your favorite herbs and enjoy.

Cauliflower and Broccoli Pie

     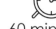

Simple   20 minutes

40 minutes   60 minutes

Ingredients:

- 1 medium head of cauliflower, florets
- 1 small head of broccoli, florets
- 6 eggs
- 1/2 cup firm tofu, crumbled
- 1/2 teaspoon nutmeg, freshly grated

Nutritional Values per Serving:

Calories   143
% Daily Value*
Total Fat 8.2g   11%
Saturated Fat 2.5g   13%
Cholesterol 279mg   93%
Sodium 135mg 6%
Total Carbohydrate 6.1g   2%
Dietary Fiber 2.5g   9%
Total Sugars 2.8g
Protein 12.5g

Directions:

1. Preheat your oven to 375 degrees F.
2. Take a large pie dish and line it with parchment paper.
3. Take a steamer basket and steam the cauliflower and broccoli florets until they are just tender, about 6 minutes. Drain it well and set it aside for further use.
4. Take a large mixing bowl and crack the eggs in it.
5. Then whisk them with crumbled tofu and freshly grated nutmeg together.
6. Stir until combined.
7. Combine the steamed cauliflower and broccoli florets with egg mixture over the vegetables and gently toss until the vegetables are evenly coated.
8. Transfer this mixture to the lined pie dish, spreading it out evenly.
9. Add it to the preheated oven and bake for 25-30 minutes.
10. Serve.

Pumpkin and Mushroom Risotto

   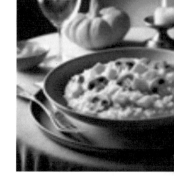

Simple   20 minutes

35 minutes   55 minutes

Ingredients:

- 1 cup arborio rice
- 2 cups pumpkin, diced into small cubes
- 1 cup mushrooms (such as cremini or button), sliced
- 4 cups low-sodium vegetable broth
- 1/2 cup low-fat ricotta cheese

Nutritional Values per Serving:

Calories   277
% Daily Value*
Total Fat 2.7g 3%
Saturated Fat 1.4g   7%
Cholesterol 8mg   3%
Sodium 101mg   4%
Total Carbohydrate 52.7g   19%
Dietary Fiber 4.8g   17%
Total Sugars 4.2g
Protein 10.6g

Directions:

1. The first step is to heat vegetable broth in a saucepan over a medium flame until it shimmers.
2. Keep the heat low during the cooking process.
3. Now, during the simmering, add pumpkins and mushrooms to it.
4. Cook both vegetables for a few minutes until they become slightly soft.
5. At this stage, add the rice.
6. Cook the rice until the texture. It will take about 18 to 20 minutes.
7. Add the low-fat recorded cheese to the desired perfection once the risotto is cooked to the desired perfection.
8. Mix the cheese with the rice and vegetables, and then serve hot. Enjoy this light and favorite recipe.

Vegetarian Fajitas

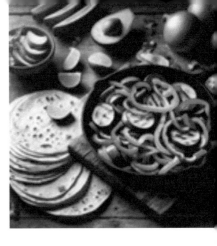

Ingredients:

- 2 bell peppers (any color), thinly sliced
- 1 large onion, thinly sliced
- 1 medium zucchini, sliced into strips
- 4 whole wheat tortillas, grilled
- 2 ripe avocados, sliced
- 2 limes cut into wedges

Simple   10 minutes   4

12 minutes   22 minutes

Nutritional Values per Serving:

Calories   260
% Daily Value*
Total Fat 11.1g   14%
Saturated Fat 2.1g   10%
Cholesterol 0mg   0%
Sodium 139mg   6%
Total Carbohydrate 39.3g   14%
Dietary Fiber 9.4g   34%
Total Sugars 5.6g
Protein 6.5g

Directions:

1. Take a skillet and heat it over medium flame.
2. Add to it onion, bell pepper, and zucchini strips
3. Sauté it for a few minutes until they are tender-crisp and slightly charred, about 8-10 minutes. Remove from heat and set aside.
4. Warm Tortillas by microwaving them for 30 minutes while covering them with damp paper towels, or grill the tortillas.
5. Now assemble the fajitas.
6. Divide the sautéed vegetables evenly among the warm tortillas.
7. Top each tortilla with sliced avocado and a squeeze of lime juice.
8. Serve:

Vegetarian Meatballs with Tomato

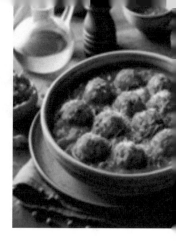

Ingredients:

Ingredients for the vegetarian meatballs:

- 2 cups cooked chickpeas, drained and rinsed
- 2 cups stale whole meal bread torn into small pieces
- 1/2 cup grated parmesan cheese
- 2 cloves garlic, minced
- 1 tablespoon chopped fresh parsley
- 1 tablespoon chopped fresh basil
- 1 teaspoon dried oregano
- pepper to taste
- 2 tablespoons olive oil for frying

For The Aromatic Herbs Tomato Sauce:

- 2 tablespoons olive oil
- 1 onion, finely chopped
- 2 cloves garlic, minced
- 1 can (14 ounces) crushed tomatoes
- 1 teaspoon dried basil
- 1 teaspoon dried oregano

Nutritional Values per Serving:

Calories   473
% Daily Value*
Total Fat 16.6g   21%
Saturated Fat 3g   15%
Cholesterol 6mg   2%
Sodium 252mg   11%
Total Carbohydrate 67.3g 24%
Dietary Fiber 16.1g 58%
Total Sugars 9.3g
Protein 22.3g

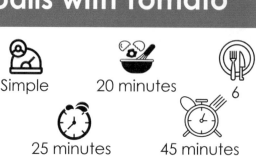

Simple   20 minutes

6

25 minutes   45 minutes

Directions:

1. First, prepare the vegetarian meatballs.
2. Take it in a food processor and add cooked chickpeas, stale whole meal bread pieces, grated Parmesan cheese, minced garlic, chopped parsley, chopped basil, dried oregano, and pepper.
3. Pulse until the mixture is combined in a fine texture.
4. Use clean hands to shape the chickpea mixture into small meatballs and add them to a baking sheet lined with parchment paper.
5. Now heat the olive oil in pan over medium flame
6. Put the meatballs into the pan in batches,
7. And cook the meatballs for about 8-10 minutes, until golden.
8. Next, transfer the meatballs to a flat plate lined with paper towels; it helps to absorb excess oil.
9. Prepare the sauce with 2 tablespoons of olive oil over medium heat.
10. Put the finely chopped onion and minced garlic sautéing for 3-4 minutes.
11. Add the crushed tomatoes, dried basil, black pepper, and dried oregano.
12. Let the sauce cook for 10-15 minutes, allowing the flavors to meld together.
13. Assembly:
14. Combine Sauce and Meatballs and simmer sauce for 5-7 minutes to heat through.
15. Serve and enjoy.

Chickpea and Spinach Stew

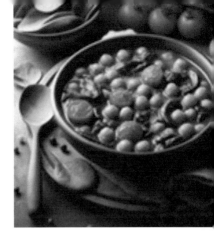

Ingredients:

- 1/2 cup cooked chickpeas
- 1 cup fresh spinach
- 1/2 cup cherry tomatoes, halved
- 1/4 onion, finely chopped
- 1/4 teaspoon ground cumin
- 1 cup low-sodium vegetable broth

 Simple   10 minutes 1

 20 minutes   30 minutes

Nutritional Values per Serving:

Calories: Approx. 250
Total Fat: 4g (5%)
Saturated Fat: 0.5g (3%)
Cholesterol: 0mg (0%)
Sodium: 300mg (13%)
Total Carbohydrates: 42g (15%)
Dietary Fiber: 12g (43%)
Total Sugars: 8g
Protein: 14g

Directions:

1. Heat a medium-sized pot over medium heat.
2. Add the chopped onion to the pot and sauté until it becomes translucent and slightly golden, about 3-5 minutes. If needed, add a bit of vegetable broth to prevent sticking.
3. Add the ground cumin and mix well with the onion, toasting the spices for about 1 minute to enhance their flavor.
4. Add the cooked chickpeas, halved cherry tomatoes, and low-sodium vegetable broth to the pot. Bring to a boil.
5. Reduce heat and let simmer for about 15 minutes, or until the cherry tomatoes start to break down and the broth has slightly reduced.
6. Add the fresh spinach and cook for another 2-3 minutes, or until the spinach has wilted and the stew has reached the desired consistency.
7. Taste and adjust salt if necessary (remembering that the DASH diet recommends limiting sodium).
8. Serve hot.

SECTION 2:

Recipes with White Meat and Hamburgers

Grilled Turkey Steak with Orzo and Arugula Salad

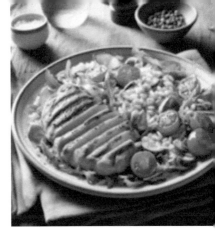

Ingredients:

- 1 turkey steak (about 150g)
- 1/2 cup pearl barley, cooked according to package instructions
- 1 cup fresh arugula
- 1/2 cup cherry tomatoes, halved
- 1/4 cucumber, thinly sliced
- 1 tablespoon extra-virgin olive oil
- 1 tablespoon balsamic vinegar
- Salt and black pepper, to taste

Nutritional Values per Serving:

Calories: Approx. 450
Total Fat: 15g (19%)
Saturated Fat: 3g (15%)
Cholesterol: 70mg (23%)
Sodium: 200mg (9%)
Total Carbohydrates: 45g (16%)
Dietary Fiber: 8g (29%)
Total Sugars: 6g
Protein: 35g

Simple   15 minutes   1
10 minutes   25 minutes

Directions:

1. Preheat the grill to medium-high heat.
2. Grill for about 4-5 minutes per side, or until well-cooked yet still juicy. Let rest for a few minutes before slicing.
3. Meanwhile, in a large bowl, combine the cooked pearl barley, arugula, halved cherry tomatoes, and cucumber slices.
4. Dress the salad with extra virgin olive oil, balsamic vinegar, and a pinch of salt. Mix well to ensure the salad is evenly dressed.
5. Arrange the salad on a serving plate. Slice the grilled turkey steak and place it on top of the salad.

Turkey Burger with Yogurt Sauce

Ingredients:

- 1 pound ground turkey
- 1 teaspoon of dill powder or more
- 4 whole wheat burger buns
- 1 cup greek yogurt
- 1 large cucumber, grated
- fresh dill, as needed

Nutritional Values per Serving:

Calories   265
% Daily Value*
Total Fat 5.9g 8%
Saturated Fat 0.9g   5%
Cholesterol 27mg   9%
Sodium 327mg   14%
Total Carbohydrate 39.9g   15%
Dietary Fiber 7.5g   27%
Total Sugars 4.4g
Protein 21.5g

Simple   20 minutes   4
10 minutes   30 minutes

Directions:

1. Squeeze excess water from grated cucumbers and set aside for further use.
2. The next step is to preheat your grill over medium-high heat.
3. Add ground turkey and dill to a large mixing bowl.
4. Mix the ingredients well and prepare a mixture for patties.
5. Use clean hands to divide the turkey mixture into equally distributed portions.
6. Then, shape each portion into patties for the burger.
7. Put the turkey patties on the preheated grill.
8. Let it grill for 4-5 minutes on each side.
9. Check with the kitchen thermometer. It gives an internal temperature of 165 degrees F.
10. Toast the buns on the grill for just a minute as well.
11. Meanwhile, let's prepare the yogurt sauce.
12. For that, take a separate bowl and add grated cucumber.
13. Add fresh dill and yogurt to it & Mix well.
14. Next, remove the patties from the grill grate and rest the patties for a minute.
15. Assemble the burgers by adding a patty on each toasted bun and topping it with a generous dollop of the yogurt dill sauce. Enjoy.

Baked Chicken with Potatoes and Rosemary

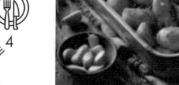

Ingredients:

- 4 chicken pieces (such as thighs or drumsticks)
- 4 medium potatoes
- Few fresh rosemary sprigs
- 4 teaspoons of rosemary, dry (divided)
- 4 cloves of garlic, minced
- 1 cup low-sodium chicken broth
-

Nutritional Values per Serving:

Calories   451
% Daily Value*
Total Fat 11.2g   14%
Saturated Fat 3.1g   16%
Cholesterol 130mg   43%
Sodium 244mg   11%
Total Carbohydrate 35.7g   13%
Dietary Fiber 5.6g   20%
Total Sugars 2.5g
Protein 48.9g

 Intermediate   20 minutes

 55 minutes   75 minutes

Directions:

1. The first step is to preheat the oven to 380 degrees Fahrenheit.
2. Next, wash the potatoes well by scrubbing them with a sponge.
3. Cut the potatoes into wedges.
4. Add the potato into a large mixing ball along with garlic and dry rosemary.
5. Next, wash and pat dry the chicken.
6. Coat the chicken well with the dried rosemary and minced garlic.
7. Then, add the chicken pieces and the potatoes to the lined baking sheet.
8. Next, add the low-sodium chicken broth over the chicken and potato inside the baking sheet.
9. This will help to keep the chicken moist.
10. Add a few rosemary springs to cover the baking sheet with aluminum foil.
11. Then, bake it in a preheated oven for about 40 minutes.
12. After 40 minutes, remove the foil from the top and continue baking with chicken and potatoes for about 15 minutes.
13. Until now, the chicken will be cooked through, and the potatoes will get tender and golden brown from the top.
14. Take the baking sheet from the oven and let it sit for a few minutes before serving.
15. Enjoy this Hearty and comforting meal

43

Chicken and Spinach Burger

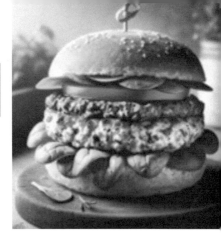

Ingredients:

- 1.5 pounds of minced chicken
- 2 cups fresh spinach, chopped
- 4 whole wheat burger buns
- 1-2 small red tomato, sliced
- 1 cup of lettuce leaves

 Intermediate

 20 minutes

 4

 15 minutes

 35 minutes

Nutritional Values per Serving:

Calories   288
% Daily Value*
Total Fat 4.1g 5%
Saturated Fat 3.4g   17%
Cholesterol 29mg   10%
Sodium 509mg   22%
Total Carbohydrate 43.1g   16%
Dietary Fiber 8.4g   30%
Total Sugars 4.9g
Protein 21.2g

Directions:

1. Add the chopped spinach and the minced chicken to a mixing bowl.
2. Stir thoroughly to incorporate the ingredients well.
3. Prepare the mixture of chicken and spinach into four equal patties.
4. Turn the heat up to medium-high on a grill or grill pan. Lightly oil sprays the pan or grill grates to prevent them from sticking.
5. Put the chicken and spinach patties onto a grill pan or grill that has already been heated.
6. Cook the patties from both sides until their internal temperature reaches 165 degrees F.
7. As the patties are cooking, get the toppings ready. Slice and clean the tomato. Clean and pat the lettuce leaves.
8. Toast the whole wheat burger buns under the grill for two minutes or until warm and lightly browned.
9. Take the patties off the grill as soon as they are fully cooked.
10. Place a chicken and spinach patty on the bottom half of each toasted burger bun to assemble the burgers. Add lettuce leaves and tomato slices to the top of each patty.
11. Place the top half of the burger buns over the burgers.
12. Serve the Chicken and Spinach Burgers immediately with your preferred condiments or side dishes. Savor this tasty and nutritious dish that fits the DASH diet!

Turkey Rolls with Ham and Sage

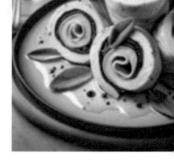

Ingredients:

- 4 turkey cutlets or turkey breast slices
- 4 slices of lean ham
- few fresh sage leaves
- 1/2 cup white wine

 Intermediate   20 minutes   4

 30 minutes   50 minutes

Nutritional Values per Serving:

Calories   287
% Daily Value*
Total Fat 7.6g 10%
Saturated Fat 2.3g   11%
Cholesterol 121mg   40%
Sodium 1131mg   49%
Total Carbohydrate 1.1g   0%
Dietary Fiber 0g   0%
Total Sugars 0.1g
Protein 48.2g

Directions:

1. First, turn your oven to 370 degrees F and preheat it for a few minutes.
2. Arrange the slices of turkey breast or cutlets on a clean work surface.
3. For each turkey cutlet, place a piece of lean ham on top.
4. Evenly distribute the fresh sage leaves across the ham pieces.
5. Depending on your taste, you can use as many or as few sage leaves as you like.
6. Roll each turkey cutlet carefully, encasing the sage and ham inside.
7. To keep the rolls together, fasten them with toothpicks or kitchen thread.
8. Add the turkey rolls to a safe, non-stick skillet to use in the oven.
9. The turkey rolls should be seared until golden brown on all sides.
10. When the turkey rolls turn brown, pour the white wine into the skillet and boil for a while.
11. After preheating the oven, move the skillet inside.
12. Bake it for about 20 to 25 minutes, or until the turkey is cooked through and, when checked with a kitchen thermometer, it reaches an internal temperature of 165 degrees F.
13. After cooking, take the skillet out of the oven.
14. Remove the string or toothpicks from the turkey rolls with caution.
15. 1. Drizzle the warm turkey rolls with sage, ham, and the skillet's white wine sauce. Serve and enjoy.

Chicken Hunter

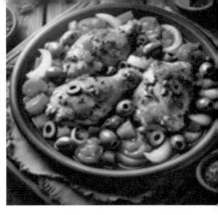

Ingredients:

- 4 chicken thighs or chicken breasts
- 2 red tomatoes, diced
- 1 white onion, diced
- 1/2 cup pitted olives (green or black), sliced
- 2 tablespoons capers
- 1 cup mixed herbs (such as thyme, rosemary, and oregano), chopped

Intermediate   15 minutes   4

30 minutes   40 minutes

Nutritional Values per Serving:

Calories   234
% Daily Value*
Total Fat 9.3g 12%
Saturated Fat 2.4g   12%
Cholesterol 89mg   30%
Sodium 1680mg   73%
Total Carbohydrate 7.3g   3%
Dietary Fiber 3.1g   11%
Total Sugars 2.5g
Protein 30.9g

Directions:

1. Turn the oven to 390 degrees F and preheat it briefly.
2. Transfer the chopped herbs, olives, capers, onions, and diced tomatoes into a mixing bowl.
3. Mix well.
4. Then, add this to a baking sheet lined with parchment paper.
5. Put the chicken breasts or thighs on top of the mixture of vegetables.
6. Fold the aluminum foil over the baking dish.
7. In a preheated oven, bake for approximately 25 to 30 minutes.
8. Take the baking dish out of the oven after the chicken is done.
9. If desired, top it with additional chopped herbs.
10. Enjoy.

BBQ Chicken Burger

Ingredients:

- 1.5 pounds of minced chicken
- 1/2 cup low-sodium bbq sauce
- 4 whole wheat burger buns
- 1 red onion, thinly sliced

Nutritional Values per Serving:

Calories 297
% Daily Value*
Total Fat 2.2g 3%
Saturated Fat 0.6g 3%
Cholesterol 29mg 10%
Sodium 515mg 22%
Total Carbohydrate 48.3g 18%
Dietary Fiber 4.5g 16%
Total Sugars 5.1g
Protein 21.2g

 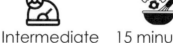

Intermediate   15 minutes   4

15 minutes   30 minutes

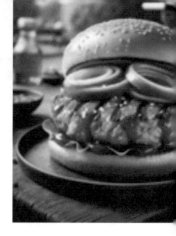

Directions:

1. Set the temperature of your grill pan or grill to medium-high.
2. Add the low-sodium BBQ sauce and the chopped chicken into a large mixing bowl.
3. Blend until thoroughly combined
4. Divide this mixture into equal portions.
5. Each piece should resemble a burger patty.
6. Cook the patties by placing them on the prepared grill or grill pan.
7. Grill the burgers on each side for 5 to 6 minutes.
8. As the burgers are cooking, get the toppings ready. Cut the red onion thinly.
9. Toast the whole wheat burger buns under the grill for one or two minutes or until warm and lightly browned.
10. Take the BBQ chicken burgers off the grill as soon as they are fully cooked.
11. Place a BBQ chicken patty on the bottom half of each toasted burger bun to assemble the burgers. Add sliced red onion on top of each patty.
12. Place the top half of the burger buns over the burgers.
13. Serve the Red Onion and BBQ Chicken Burgers immediately with your preferred side dishes. Savor your succulent and savory barbecued chicken burgers!

SECTION 3:

Fish and Hamburger Recipes

Salmon Burger with Coleslaw

Ingredients:

- 1.5-pound minced salmon
- ½ cup slices whole wheat bread (breadcrumbs)
- 1.5 cups cabbage (shredded)
- 1/2 cup greek yogurt, low-fat
- 2 tablespoons dill (chopped), divided
- 4 slices of whole wheat bread, toasted

Nutritional Values per Serving:

Calories 278
% Daily Value*
Total Fat 7.1g 9%
Saturated Fat 1.5g 7%
Cholesterol 34mg 11%
Sodium 321mg 14%
Total Carbohydrate 29g 11%
Dietary Fiber 5.8g 21%
Total Sugars 6.5g
Protein 25.5g

Simple   10 minutes

10 minutes   20 minutes

Directions:

1. Add whole wheat breadcrumbs, dill, and salmon in a large mixing bowl.
2. Mix everything until thoroughly combined.
3. Shape the salmon mixture into patties for burgers.
4. Take a skillet and heat it over medium flame
5. Then the skillet should be non-stick
6. Put the salmon patties into the skillet and let it cook for 4-5 minutes on each side.
7. Once brown and crispy from all sides, it's done.
8. Meanwhile, prepare coleslaw to serve with the burger by adding cabbage, yogurt, and dill to a bowl and mixing well.
9. Serve the cooked salmon burgers on whole wheat buns with coleslaw.
10. Enjoy.

Baked Sea Bass Fillets with Olives and Capers

Ingredients:

- 2 (6 ounces each) sea bass fillets
- ½ cup of olives (pitted)
- 1/3 cup of capers
- little lemon (sliced)

Nutritional Values per Serving:

Calories 133
% Daily Value*
Total Fat 6.8g 9%
Saturated Fat 1.4g 7%
Cholesterol 15mg 5%
Sodium 962mg 42%
Total Carbohydrate 14.4g 5%
Dietary Fiber 1.3g 5%
Total Sugars 1.1g
Protein 5.6g

Simple   10 minutes

20 minutes   30 minutes

Directions:

1. Preheat the oven to 350 degrees F.
2. Take a large baking dish and line it with parchment paper.
3. Place the sea bass fillets onto the lined baking dish.
4. Put the olives and capers beside the sea bass fillets.
5. Arrange lemon slices on top of fish fillets.
6. Cover the baking dish with aluminum foil.
7. Next, bake it in the oven for 15-20 minutes.
8. Remove and serve with chopped herbs if you like.

Tuna Burger with Wasabi Mayonnaise

Ingredients:

- 1 pound of ground tuna
- 1 whole wheat bread (crumbled into breadcrumbs)
- 1 tablespoon wasabi
- 1/3 cup of low-fat mayonnaise
- 4 whole wheat bread slices, toasted

 Simple 8minutes   4

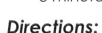 8 minutes   16 minutes

Nutritional Values per Serving:

Calories   268
% Daily Value*
Total Fat 7.8g 10%
Saturated Fat 1.1g   6%
Cholesterol 27mg   9%
Sodium 477mg   21%
Total Carbohydrate 33.1g   12%
Dietary Fiber 6.8g   24%
Total Sugars 3.4g
Protein 17.8g

Directions:

1. Add ground tuna and crumbled whole wheat bread in a large mixing bowl.
2. Mix the ingredients well and shape them into burger patties.
3. Take a medium-sized non-stick skillet and heat it over a medium flame.
4. Then, add the patties to the skillet.
5. Cook the patties for 4 minutes per side.
6. Meanwhile, prepare the wasabi mayonnaise by mixing the wasabi into the low-fat mayonnaise mix well for a fine consistency.
7. When the tuna patties are cooked, serve them on whole wheat bread slices
8. Top it with prepared wasabi mayonnaise and serve.

Teriyaki Salmon with Brown Rice

Ingredients:

- 2 salmon fillets
- 4 teaspoons of low sodium teriyaki sauce
- 2 cups cooked brown rice
- 2 teaspoons of sesame seeds (for garnish)

 Simple 10 minutes 2

 8 minutes   18 minutes

Nutritional Values per Serving:

% Daily Value*
Total Fat 24.5g   31%
Saturated Fat 4.1g   21%
Cholesterol 90mg   30%
Sodium 519mg   23%
Total Carbohydrate 49.1g   18%
Dietary Fiber 1.3g   5%
Total Sugars 5.6g
Protein 44.2g

Directions:

1. First, turn the oven to 375 degrees F to preheat for a few minutes.
2. Stir together the low-sodium teriyaki sauce and coat the fish fillets with it. Adjust the amount of sauce to your taste.
3. Add the salmon to the baking sheet lined with parchment paper and bake it in the preheated oven for 12 minutes.
4. Cook the salmon until it gets flakey.
5. Add the salmon over cooked brown rice and serve it hot with a garnish of sesame seeds.

Cod Burger with Tartar Sauce

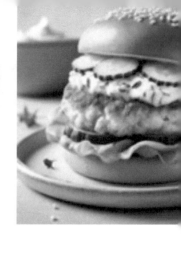

Ingredients:

- 2 pounds of cod fillet, ground
- 1 cup whole wheat bread (crumbled into breadcrumbs)
- few pickled cucumbers
- 1 cup of greek yogurt

Nutritional Values per Serving:

Calories   266
% Daily Value*
Total Fat 3.6g 5%
Saturated Fat 1.3g   7%
Cholesterol 58mg   19%
Sodium 330mg   14%
Total Carbohydrate 22.7g 8%
Dietary Fiber 3.4g   12%
Total Sugars 4.8g
Protein 34.4g

Simple   10 minutes
10 minutes   20 minutes   2

Directions:

1. Take a large mixing bowl and add ground cod to it.
2. Then add crumbled whole wheat bread
3. Mix the ingredients well:
4. Shape the cod mixture into patties.
5. Take a medium-sized non-stick skillet and heat it over medium flame.
6. Add the .cod patties to the skillet and cook for about 4-5 minutes on each side,
7. Meanwhile, prepare the tartar sauce; take a small bowl and add pickled cucumbers with Greek yogurt to create the tartar sauce.
8. Adjust the proportions of pickled cucumbers and Greek yogurt according to your liking.
9. Once the cod patties are cooked, serve them on whole wheat buns (optional) with a dollop of the prepared tartar sauce on top.

Grilled Sea bream With Mediterranean Salad

Ingredients:

- 2 (6 ounces each) Sea Bream fillets
- Salad ingredients
- few cherry tomatoes
- 1 cup of red onion
- few olives, or as needed
- few slices of cucumbers, or as needed

Nutritional Values per Serving:

Calories   231
% Daily Value*
Total Fat 11.2g   14%
Saturated Fat 2.6g   13%
Cholesterol 31mg   10%
Sodium 486mg   21%
Total Carbohydrate 20.1g 7%
Dietary Fiber 1.5g   5%
Total Sugars 2.1g
Protein 13.9g

Simple   6 minutes
6 minutes   12 minutes   2

Directions:

1. Set your grill temperature to medium-high.
2. Add the sea's bream fillet to the grill grate and let it grill for 3 minutes per side.
3. Transfer the sea bream fillets to a plate when they are cooked and have grill marks.
4. Diced cucumbers, red onion, olives, and cherry tomato slices
5. Add them to a large mixing bowl.
6. Mix the salad ingredients until thoroughly blended.
7. Once the sea bream fillets are cooked, serve them hot alongside the prepared delicious salad.
8. Enjoy.

Shrimp Burger with Avocado

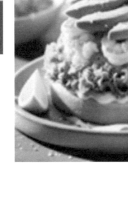

Ingredients:

- 1 pound ground shrimp
- 4 slices whole wheat bread (crumbled into breadcrumbs)
- 1 avocado (sliced)
- ½ cup of chopped lettuce leaves
- lime wedges (for serving)

Nutritional Values per Serving:

Calories   416
% Daily Value*
Total Fat 13.6g   17%
Saturated Fat 2.5g   12%
Cholesterol 155mg   52%
Sodium 1168mg   51%
Total Carbohydrate 35.2g   13%
Dietary Fiber 8.7g   31%
Total Sugars 6.3g
Protein 42.6g

 Simple
 10 minutes
 2
 8 minutes
 18 minutes

Directions:

1. Add the ground shrimp with whole wheat bread crumbs in a large mixing bowl.
2. Mix them well for a pleasing combination.
3. Divide this prepared mixture into four equal portions.
4. Shape the mixture into patties.
5. Heat a non-stick skillet and heat it over medium flame
6. Next, place the patties onto the skillet.
7. Cook for 3-4 minutes on each side.
8. Meanwhile, prepare the avocado slices and lettuce leaves.
9. Once the patties are ready, assemble the burgers by layering a lettuce leaf on the bottom of the whole wheat bun, followed by a shrimp patty, and then topping it with avocado slices.
10. Serve and enjoy.

CHAPTER 8:

SNACKS

Vegetable Sticks with Hummus

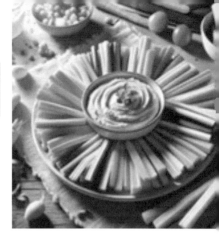

Ingredients:

- 2 large carrots cut into sticks
- 2 stalks of celery cut into sticks
- 2 green bell peppers cut into strips
- 2 yellow bell peppers cut into strips
- 1 cup hummus

Nutritional Values per Serving:

Calories   302
% Daily Value*
Total Fat 12.5g 16%
Saturated Fat 1.8g   9%
Cholesterol 0mg   0%
Sodium 626mg 27%
Total Carbohydrate 39.7g   14%
Dietary Fiber 13.2g   47%
Total Sugars 12.3g
Protein 12.6g

Simple   15 minutes   2

0 minutes   15 minutes

Directions:

1. First wash the veggie.
2. Then cut the peppers, celery, and carrots into strips.
3. Place the veggie sticks in serving tray or plate for serving.
4. Place hummus beside the veggies and serve.

Greek Yogurt with Honey and Nuts

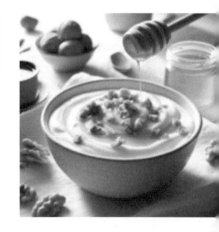

Ingredients:

- 1.5 cups of low-fat greek yogurt
- 2 tablespoons honey, more to taste
- 4 tablespoons walnuts, chopped

Nutritional Values per Serving:

Calories   156
% Daily Value*
Total Fat 6.7g 9%
Saturated Fat 0.7g   4%
Cholesterol 3mg   1%
Sodium 27mg   1%
Total Carbohydrate 21.9g 8%
Dietary Fiber 0.7g   3%
Total Sugars 20.9g
Protein 4.5g

Simple   10 minutes   3

0 minutes   10 minutes

Directions:

1. Spoon the low-fat Greek yogurt into a serving bowl or individual cups.
2. Pour the honey over the yogurt.
3. Top it with nuts at the end
4. Serve and enjoy.

Fresh Fruit with Almond Butter

Ingredients:

- 2 apples, sliced
- 2 pears, sliced
- 2 tablespoons almond butter

Nutritional Values per Serving:

Calories   224
% Daily Value*
Total Fat 5.3g 7%
Saturated Fat 0.5g   2%
Cholesterol 0mg   0%
Sodium 39mg   2%
Total Carbohydrate 47.7g   17%
Dietary Fiber 8.8g   31%
Total Sugars 33.3g
Protein 2.2g

Simple   5 minutes

 2

0 minutes   5 minutes

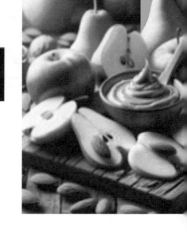

Directions:

1. Wash the apples and pears, and then slice them into thin wedges or rounds.
2. Arrange the sliced fruit on a serving plate.
3. Place the almond butter in a small bowl.
4. Serve the fresh fruit alongside the almond butter for dipping.
5. Dip the fruit slices into the almond butter and enjoy the delicious and healthy snack.

Baked Apple Chips > Apples, Cinnamon.

Ingredients:

- 1 large apple
- 1/2 teaspoon ground cinnamon

Simple   10 minutes

2

2 hours   2 hours and 10 minutes

Nutritional Values per Serving:

Calories: Approx. 95
Total Fat: 0.3g (0%)
Saturated Fat: 0g (0%)
Cholesterol: 0mg (0%)
Sodium: 2mg (0%)
Total Carbohydrates: 25g (9%)
Dietary Fiber: 4.4g (16%)
Total Sugars: 19g
Protein: 0.5g

Directions:

1. Preheat the oven to 95°C (200°F). Line a baking sheet with parchment paper.
2. Wash and dry the apple. Core and slice the apple into thin slices, about 1/8 inch thick.
3. Arrange the apple slices in a single layer on the prepared baking sheet. Evenly sprinkle with ground cinnamon.
4. Bake in the preheated oven for about 1 hour. Flip the apple slices and continue to bake for another hour, or until the chips are dry and the edges start to curl up slightly. Baking time may vary depending on the thickness of the slices and the type of apple used.
5. Turn off the oven and let the apple chips inside until the oven has completely cooled, to help them get even crispier.
6. Remove the apple chips from the oven and let them cool completely before serving.

Mini Whole Wheat Bread Sandwich with Avocado and Turkey

Ingredients:

- 12 slices whole wheat bread
- 1 large ripe avocado
- 12 slices turkey breast

Nutritional Values per Serving:

Calories   380
% Daily Value*
Total Fat 8.5g 11%
Saturated Fat 1.8g   9%
Cholesterol 86mg   29%
Sodium 2295mg   100%
Total Carbohydrate 33g   12%
Dietary Fiber 5.9g   21%
Total Sugars 10.2g
Protein 41.7g

Simple   15 minutes   6

0 minutes   15 minutes

Directions:

1. Cut the avocado in half and remove the pits.
2. Transfer the flesh of avocados into a small mixing bowl.
3. Next, mash the avocado using a fork.
4. Toast the whole wheat bread pieces until they are lightly brown and crispy.
5. Place a generous amount of mashed avocado onto toasted bread slices.
6. Put the 2 slices of turkey breast into each slice of bread and spread with avocado.
7. Prepare the sandwiches and place another slice of toasted whole wheat bread on each.
8. Slice each sandwich and once all the sandwiches are ready, serve.

Banana and Oat Muffins

Ingredients:

- 2 fully matured bananas, thoroughly crushed
- 1 cup of oats
- 2 eggs
- 2 teaspoons of honey

Nutritional Values per Serving:

Calories   394
% Daily Value*
Total Fat 8g   10%
Saturated Fat 2.1g   11%
Cholesterol 186mg   62%
Sodium 74mg   3%
Total Carbohydrate 72.1g 26%
Dietary Fiber 7.2g   26%
Total Sugars 32.5g
Protein 13g

Simple   10 minutes   2

20 minutes   30 minutes

Directions:

1. Set your oven to a temperature of 350 degrees F before using it.
2. Line muffin cups with muffin papers.
3. Using a fork, thoroughly crush the ripe bananas in a mixing dish until they reach a smooth consistency.
4. Combine the oats, eggs, and honey with the mashed bananas. Thoroughly blend the items until they are fully incorporated.
5. Transfer this muffin batter into the prepared muffin tin, ensuring that each cup is filled to about two-thirds of its capacity.
6. Cook in the prepared oven for 18-20 minutes.
7. Remove the muffins from the oven once done, and let them cool.
8. Serve and savor these nutritious Banana and Oat Muffins.

Whole Wheat Crackers with Fresh Cheese and Tomatoes

Ingredients:

- 10 whole wheat crackers
- cream cheese (or any fresh cheese of your choice)
- few cherry tomatoes, halved

Nutritional Values per Serving:

Calories 176
% Daily Value*
Total Fat 13.9g 18%
Saturated Fat 7.8g 39%
Cholesterol 37mg 12%
Sodium 187mg 8%
Total Carbohydrate 10g 4%
Dietary Fiber 1.4g 5%
Total Sugars 0.1g
Protein 3.7g

Simple   15 minutes   3

0 minutes   15 minutes

Directions:

1. Place the whole wheat crackers organized on a serving platter or plate.
2. Apply a thin coating of cream cheese onto each cracker.
3. Position one cherry tomato half on the cheese layer of each cracker.
4. Continue the process iteratively until all crackers are garnished with cheese and tomatoes.
5. Serve promptly and savor the delectable amalgamation of flavors and textures.

Dried Fruit and Seeds

Ingredients:

- 1/2 cup almonds
- 1/2 cup walnuts
- 1/4 cup pumpkin seeds
- 1/4 cup sunflower seeds

Simple   5 minutes   2

0 minutes   5 minutes

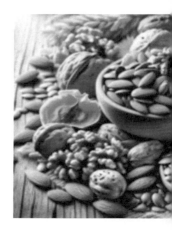

Directions:

1. Combine the almonds, walnuts, pumpkin seeds, and sunflower seeds in a mixing dish.
2. Place the assortment of dried fruit and seeds into a container or divide them into separate snack bags for easy access.

Nutritional Values per Serving:

Calories 471
% Daily Value*
Total Fat 42.5g 54%
Saturated Fat 3.6g 18%
Cholesterol 0mg 0%
Sodium 4mg 0%
Total Carbohydrate 12.9g 5%
Dietary Fiber 6.7g 24%
Total Sugars 1.8g
Protein 18.2g

Homemade Energy Bars

Ingredients:

- 1 cup rolled oats
- 1/3 cup dried fruits
- 2 tablespoons chia seeds
- 1/4 cup honey
- 1/2 cup peanut butter

Nutritional Values per Serving:

Calories 343
% Daily Value*
Total Fat 10.6g   14%
Saturated Fat 2.1g   11%
Cholesterol 0mg   0%
Sodium 86mg   4%
Total Carbohydrate 56.7g 21%
Dietary Fiber 7.1g   25%
Total Sugars 19.4g
Protein 9.9g

 Easy
 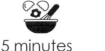 5 minutes

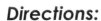 0 minutes
 3 15 minutes

Directions:

1. Combine the rolled oats, dried fruits, and chia seeds in a large mixing dish.
2. Mix honey with peanut butter in a small saucepan and let it warm over a low flame.
3. Transfer the honey-peanut butter mixture to the dry ingredients in the mixing bowl.
4. Continuously stir the mixture until all components are combined.
5. Cover the inside of a baking dish or pan with parchment paper, ensuring extra paper extends beyond the edges for convenient removal.
6. Transfer this prepared mixture to the lined baking dish.
7. Refrigerate the baking dish for at least 1 hour or until the mixture has solidified and become firm.
8. After the mixture has been set, please remove it from the refrigerator and use a keen knife to slice it into rectangular or square shapes. Enjoy.

Berry & Spinach Smoothie

Ingredients:

- 1 cup mixed berries
- 1-1/2 cup fresh spinach leaves
- 1/2 cup low-fat greek yogurt
- 1/2 cup almond milk

Nutritional Values per Serving:

Calories 82
% Daily Value*
Total Fat 4.4g 6%
Saturated Fat 3.7g   18%
Cholesterol 1mg   0%
Sodium 38mg   2%
Total Carbohydrate 9.3g   3%
Dietary Fiber 2.3g   8%
Total Sugars 6.2g
Protein 2.2g

 Simple
 5 minutes

 0 minutes
 3 5 minutes

Directions:

1. Wash the spinach leaves and berries.
2. Blend the almond milk, Greek yogurt, fresh spinach leaves, mixed berries, and spinach in a high-speed blender.
3. Serve right away by pouring the smoothie into the ice-filled serving glasses.

Air Popcorn without Salt

Ingredients:
- 2 cups air-popped popcorn
- a pinch of paprika

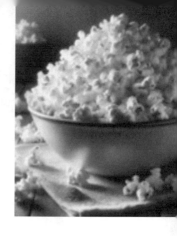

Easy   5 minutes   2

5 minutes   10 minutes

Nutritional Values per Serving:
Calories   209
% Daily Value*
Total Fat 11.3g   14%
Saturated Fat 1.8g   9%
Cholesterol 0mg   0%
Sodium 133mg   6%
Total Carbohydrate 32.8g   12%
Dietary Fiber 19.6g   70%
Total Sugars 5.2g
Protein 8.2g

Directions:
1. Follow the manufacturer's directions to prepare air-popped popcorn.
2. Place the recently popped popcorn in a big basin.
3. After gently tossing the popcorn to coat, sprinkle a pinch of paprika.
4. Enjoy the crisp, savory flavor of Air Popcorn without Salt immediately/.

Cucumbers Stuffed with Ricotta and Herbs

Ingredients:
- 2 cucumbers
- 1/2 cup ricotta cheese
- 4 tablespoons chopped fresh mixed herbs
- freshly ground black pepper, to taste

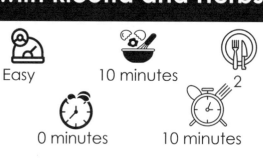
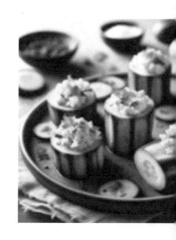

Easy   10 minutes   2

0 minutes   10 minutes

Nutritional Values per Serving:
Calories   50
% Daily Value*
Total Fat 2.1g 3%
Saturated Fat 1.3g   6%
Cholesterol 8mg   3%
Sodium 33mg   1%
Total Carbohydrate 4.9g   2%
Dietary Fiber 0.5g   2%
Total Sugars 1.8g
Protein 3.5g

Directions:
1. Before using, wash the cucumbers thoroughly.
2. Then pat dry cucumber with paper towel.
3. Cut the cucumbers in half lengthwise and then into even slices, approximately 2 inches each.
4. Carefully hollow out the core of each cucumber by using a small spoon or melon baller to scrape out the seeds, reserving around 1/4 inch of flesh.
5. Mix the ricotta cheese and the fresh herbs in a bowl.
6. After you hollow out each cucumber segment, fill it up to the top with the ricotta mixture using a spoon.
7. Place the cucumbers that have been filled with filling on a serving dish.
8. Season it with freshly ground black pepper.
9. Once ready, dig in.

Baked Kale Chips

Ingredients:
- 1 bunch kale
- 1 tablespoon olive oil
- 1/2 teaspoon smoked paprika

Nutritional Values per Serving:

Calories 49
% Daily Value*
Total Fat 0g 0%
Saturated Fat 0g 0%
Cholesterol 0mg 0%
Sodium 43mg 2%
Total Carbohydrate 10.5g 4%
Dietary Fiber 1.5g 5%
Total Sugars 0g
Protein 3g

 Easy   10 minutes   2

 15 minutes 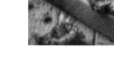 25 minutes

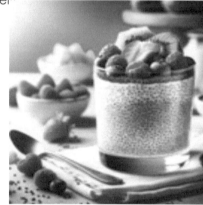

Directions:
1. Get your oven ready for 300 degrees F.
2. Line a baking sheet with parchment paper.
3. Remove excess water from the kale leaves and dry them with a paper towel.
4. After removing the rough stems, chop the kale leaves into small pieces.
5. Toss the kale, olive oil, and smoked paprika in a large mixing basin.
6. Lay the kale pieces on the baking sheet.
7. Bake for 10 to 15 minutes or until the kale chips are crunchy and beginning to get a little golden brown.
8. To avoid burning, check on the kale chips after the baking time is almost up.
9. Let the kale chips cool on the baking sheet after taking them out of the oven.
10. Serve the Baked Kale Chips immediately.

Chia Pudding

Ingredients:
- 1/4 cup chia seeds
- 6 ounces of coconut milk
- 1/2 teaspoon vanilla extract
- Fresh fruit (mixed berries or kiwi)

 Easy 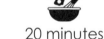 20 minutes   2

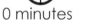 0 minutes   20 minutes

Nutritional Values per Serving:

Calories 365
% Daily Value*
Total Fat 29.7g 38%
Saturated Fat 25.5g 127%
Cholesterol 0mg 0%
Sodium 21mg 1%
Total Carbohydrate 11.3g 4%
Dietary Fiber 3.9g 14%
Total Sugars 7.2g
Protein 3.4g

Directions:
1. Blend the chia seeds, coconut milk, and vanilla essence in a container or basin. Make sure the chia seeds are dispersed evenly by stirring well.
2. Cover the bowl and refrigerate it for at least 2-4 hours.
3. Stir or shake the mixture occasionally while refrigerated to avoid clumping.
4. Take the chia pudding out of the fridge when it has set.
5. Layer the chia pudding with fresh fruit in miniature glasses or jars to make the Jars of Chia Pudding.
6. Serve.

Mini Spinach and Feta Quiche

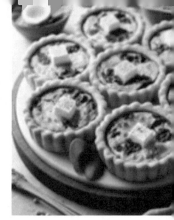

Ingredients:

- 2 cups of chopped fresh spinach
- ½ cup of feta cheese, crumbled
- 4 eggs
- 1/3 teaspoon of nutmeg

Easy   10 minutes

20 minutes   30 minutes   2

Nutritional Values per Serving:

Calories   232
% Daily Value*
Total Fat 15.7g   20%
Saturated Fat 6.9g   35%
Cholesterol 394mg   131%
Sodium 498mg   22%
Total Carbohydrate 5.4g   2%
Dietary Fiber 2.2g   8%
Total Sugars 2.2g
Protein 19g

Directions:

1. Before using your oven, set it to 375 degrees F.
2. Line a muffin tray with muffin liners to cover it.
3. Combine the eggs in a mixing bowl and vigorously whisk them until thoroughly beaten.
4. Incorporate the diced spinach, fragmented feta cheese, nutmeg, and salt into the eggs. Continuously mix the components until they are thoroughly and uniformly blended.
5. Distribute the egg mixture evenly across the muffin pans, ensuring that each cup is filled to about two-thirds of its capacity.
6. Cook in the oven preheated oven for 18-20 minutes.
7. Once done, allow them to cool within the muffin tray.
8. Serve.

CHAPTER 9:

SWEET & DESSERT

Chocolate Avocado Mousse

Ingredients:

- 1/2 ripe avocado
- 2 tablespoons cocoa powder
- 1 tablespoon honey (or more, to taste)
- 1/4 cup unsweetened almond milk
- 1/2 teaspoon vanilla extract

Nutritional Values per Serving:

Calories: Approx. 320
Total Fat: 19g (24%)
Saturated Fat: 3g (15%)
Cholesterol: 0mg (0%)
Sodium: 40mg (2%)
Total Carbohydrates: 37g (13%)
Dietary Fiber: 10g (36%)
Total Sugars: 22g
Protein: 5g

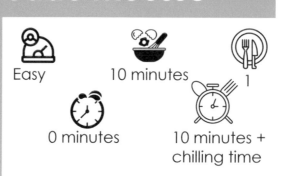

Easy   10 minutes   1

0 minutes   10 minutes + chilling time

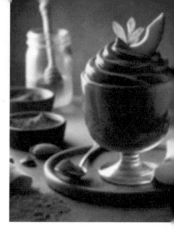

Directions:

1. Cut the avocado in half, remove the seed, and scoop out the pulp with a spoon.
2. In a blender or food processor, combine the avocado pulp, cocoa powder, honey, almond milk, and vanilla extract.
3. Blend on high speed until smooth and homogeneous, scraping the sides of the blender as necessary to ensure all ingredients are well combined.
4. Taste and adjust sweetness, adding more honey if desired.
5. Transfer the mousse to a glass or dessert cup and refrigerate for at least 1 hour, or until it has cooled and slightly set.
6. Serve cold, optionally garnished with a dusting of cocoa powder or fresh fruit as desired.

Almond Flour and Dark Chocolate Biscuits

Ingredients:

- 2 cups almond flour
- 1/2 cup dark chocolate pieces
- 2 eggs
- 1 teaspoon vanilla extract
- 1/4 cup maple syrup

Nutritional Values per Serving:

Calories   336
% Daily Value*
Total Fat 24g 31%
Saturated Fat 4.1g   20%
Cholesterol 372mg   124%
Sodium 141mg   6%
Total Carbohydrate 15.2g 6%
Dietary Fiber 3g   11%
Total Sugars 9.2g
Protein 18.6g

Simple   10 minutes   2

12 minutes   22 minutes

Directions:

1. Preheat your oven to a temperature of 350 degrees F before using it.
2. Line a baking sheet with parchment paper.
3. Combine the almond flour, dark chocolate bits, eggs, vanilla essence, and maple syrup in a mixing dish. Blend until well incorporated.
4. Take a cookie scoop to transfer the dough and place it onto the baking sheet/
5. Gently compress each biscuit using the side of a spoon.
6. Add the dough to the oven and bake for 12 minutes or until the biscuits are slightly golden brown on the edges.
7. Take the biscuits out of the oven.
8. Allow them to cool.
9. After allowing them to cool, serve, and savor these delectable Almond Flour and Dark Chocolate Biscuits as a delightful indulgence or snack.

Chia Pudding with Chocolate

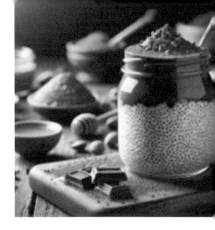

Ingredients:

- 4 tablespoons of chia seeds
- 1 cup of almond milk
- 2 tablespoons ground chocolate
- 1/2 cup honey
- 1/4 teaspoon of vanilla flavoring

 Simple   10 minutes   2

 0 minutes   10 minutes

Nutritional Values per Serving:

Calories   310
% Daily Value*
Total Fat 8.9g 11%
Saturated Fat 5.1g   25%
Cholesterol 0mg   0%
Sodium 65mg   3%
Total Carbohydrate 60.3g 22%
Dietary Fiber 0.7g   3%
Total Sugars 55.2g
Protein 2.6a

Directions:

1. Add the almond milk, chai seeds, chocolate powder, honey, and vanilla extract to a large bowl.
2. Mix all of the ingredients well.
3. Cover the bowl and put it in the fridge for at least 2 hours.
4. Ensure the pudding is well combined by stirring it thoroughly before serving.
5. Serve and enjoy.

Fruit Tart with Date and Walnut Base

Ingredients:

- 1 cup of dates without pits
- 1 cup of walnuts

Fruit topping:
- Various ripe fruits, such as berries, sliced kiwi, sliced peaches, or any other fruits you prefer.
- Greek yogurt for topping

 Simple   20 minutes 2

 0 minutes 20 minutes

Nutritional Values per Serving:

Calories   379
% Daily Value*
Total Fat 29.6g   38%
Saturated Fat 1.7g   8%
Cholesterol 0mg   0%
Sodium 2mg 0%
Total Carbohydrate 23.6g 9%
Dietary Fiber 5.4g   19%
Total Sugars 16.3g
Protein 12.6g

Directions:

1. Begin by preparing the Date and Walnut Base:
2. Blend the pitted dates and walnuts in a food processor.
3. Blend the ingredients until they combine into a cohesive.
4. Line a tart pan with butter paper.
5. Apply pressure to insert the mixture into the base of the Tart Pan firmly:
6. Place the date and walnut mixture into a tart pan.
7. Utilize your hand or thumb to apply pressure to the mixture, ensuring it is distributed uniformly around the base and edges of the tart pan, thus creating a crust.
8. Place the tart pan in the refrigerator to cool while you prepare the fruit topping.
9. Make the Fruit Topping:
10. Clean and ready your various fresh fruits. Cut or dice them according to your preference.
11. Construct the tart:
12. Take it out after the date and let the walnut base cool in the refrigerator.
13. Place the freshly prepared fruits atop the cooled
14. Place small portions of Greek yogurt on top of the fruit tart
15. Divide the fruit tart into individual portions and serve it cold.

Banana and Oat Pancakes

Ingredients:

- 2 large bananas, frozen and sliced
- 1/2 teaspoon vanilla extract
- 1/4 cup unsweetened almond milk

Nutritional Values per Serving:

Calories: Approx. 210
Total Fat: 1g (1%)
Saturated Fat: 0g (0%)
Cholesterol: 0mg (0%)
Sodium: 40mg (2%)
Total Carbohydrates: 51g (19%)
Dietary Fiber: 6g (21%)
Total Sugars: 28g
Protein: 2g

     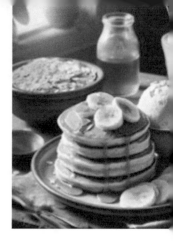

Easy   5 minutes   1
0 minutes   5 minutes

Directions:

1. Before proceeding with the recipe, ensure the bananas have been frozen for at least 2-3 hours or until they are completely solid.
2. In a blender or food processor, add the frozen banana slices, vanilla extract, and almond milk.
3. Blend on high speed until the mixture becomes smooth and creamy, similar to ice cream consistency. You may need to stop and scrape the sides of the blender occasionally to ensure all ingredients are well mixed.
4. If the ice cream is too thick, add a little more almond milk, a tablespoon at a time, until you reach the desired consistency.
5. Serve immediately for a soft ice cream or transfer to a suitable container and freeze for 1-2 hours for a firmer ice cream.
6. 1. Garnish as desired with fresh fruit, chopped nuts, or a drizzle of honey before serving.

Mango and Lime Sorbet

Ingredients:

- 2 ripe mangos cut into small pieces
- 2 limes, zest
- 3/4 cup of honey (or more or less)
- 1/2 cup of water

Nutritional Values per Serving:

Calories   90
% Daily Value*
Total Fat 0.6g 1%
Saturated Fat 0.1g   1%
Cholesterol 0mg   0%
Sodium 3mg 0%
Total Carbohydrate 25.5g 9%
Dietary Fiber 4.4g   16%
Total Sugars 15.4g
Protein 1.5g

    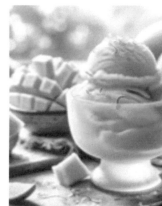

Simple   30 minutes   2
0 minutes   30 minutes

Directions:

1. Mix the mango chunks, lime zest, honey, and water in a blender or food processor.
2. To make mango puree, blend all ingredients until smooth.
3. Place the mango puree in a small, shallow bowl.
4. Cover the mixture in the fridge for at least an hour or two until it's completely cooled. T:
5. Pour the chilled mango mixture into an ice cream machine.
6. Once the mixture achieves a consistency similar to sorbet, it's done.
7. It usually takes around twenty to twenty-five minutes.
8. Divide the lime and mango sorbet among serving dishes.
9. Toss in some extra lime zest or mint leaves for garnish.

Avocado Chocolate Brownies

Ingredients:

- 1 ripe avocado
- 1/2 cups of cocoa powder
- 2 large eggs
- 1/2 cup of coconut sugar
- 1 teaspoon of vanilla extract

 Simple 15 minutes

 20 minutes 35 minutes

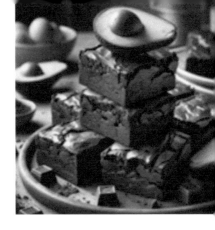

Nutritional Values per Serving:

Nutrition Facts per Servings
Calories   383
% Daily Value*
Total Fat 17.3g   22%
Saturated Fat 5.6g   28%
Cholesterol 372mg   124%
Sodium 149mg   6%
Total Carbohydrate 22.8g   8%
Dietary Fiber 9g   32%
Total Sugars 7.5g
Protein 17.6g

Directions:

1. Before using the oven, preheat it to 350 degrees F.
2. Line the parchment paper with an 8x8-inch baking pan.
3. Remove the skin and seed from the ripe avocado, and then crush it in a mixing bowl until it becomes smooth.
4. Combine the cocoa powder, eggs, coconut sugar, and vanilla essence with the mashed avocado.
5. Blend thoroughly until all ingredients are fully incorporated and the batter has a smooth consistency.
6. Transfer the batter to the prepped baking pan and distribute it evenly.
7. Cook in the oven for 20-25 minutes, or until the brownies are firm on the sides and a toothpick inserted into the center comes out with slightly wet crumbs.
8. Let the brownies cool for approximately 10 minutes.
9. Serve.

Apple and Raspberry Crumble

Ingredients:

- 4 large apples, peeled, cored, and sliced
- 1 cup raspberries
- 2-4 tablespoons honey
ingredients for the crumble topping:
- 1 cup oat flakes
- 1/3 cup ground almonds
- 4 tablespoons honey

 Simple  15 minutes

 30 minutes 45 minutes

Nutritional Values per Serving:

Calories   275
% Daily Value*
Total Fat 5.2g 7%
Saturated Fat 0.6g   3%
Cholesterol 0mg   0%
Sodium 3mg 0%
Total Carbohydrate 54.5g   20%
Dietary Fiber 8.4g   30%
Total Sugars 29.4g
Protein 5.9g

Directions:

1. First step is to preheat your oven to 350 degrees F.
2. Take a large baking sheet and line it with butter paper.
3. Take a large mixing bowl and add the sliced apples and raspberries.
4. Pour the honey over the fruit and toss it well.
5. Layer the fruit mixture onto the prepared baking dish.
6. Combine the oat flakes and ground almonds in another medium-sized mixing bowl.
7. Drizzle the honey over the mixture.
8. Stir the mixture well so it forms a crumbly texture.
9. Put the crumble topping evenly over the fruit filling inside the baking dish.
10. Place teh baking dish inside the oven and bake it for 30 minutes.
11. Once done, serve

Natural Fruit Jelly

Ingredients:

- 2 cups of 100% pure fruit juice (orange, apple, or mixed)
- 1/4 cup of gelatin powder
- (optional) slices or pieces of fresh fruit to garnish

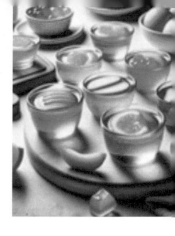

Simple   20 minutes   2

0 minutes   20 minutes

Nutritional Values per Serving:

Calories   252
% Daily Value*
Total Fat 0.3g 0%
Saturated Fat 0g   0%
Cholesterol 0mg   0%
Sodium 30mg   1%
Total Carbohydrate 67.2g 24%
Dietary Fiber 1g   4%
Total Sugars 66.2g
Protein 1.9g

Directions:

1. Pour the natural fruit juice in a saucepan and warm it over medium heat.
2. Do not boil the juice.
3. Next put the gelatin powder to the hot liquid and stir well.
4. Keep stirring the mixture constantly after the gelatin has dissolved.
5. After the gelatin dissolves, turn off flame.
6. Pour this mixture carefully into the molds.
7. You can garnish the bottom of the molds with fresh fruit slices or pieces before pouring the liquid mixture on top.
8. Put the dishes or molds into the refrigerator for 2-4 hours.
9. Take the jelly out of the fridge once it sets

Light Cheesecake with Berries

Ingredients:
- 1 cup of whole wheat biscuits, crumbled
- 2 tablespoons of almond butter

to make the cheesecake filling:
- 1 cup of ricotta cheese, low fat
- 1 cup of Greek yogurt
- 2 teaspoons of honey

ingredients for the topping:
- berries, including strawberries, blueberries, and raspberries
- 1 cup vegan jelly

Simple   25 minutes   2

40 minutes   65 minutes

Nutritional Values per Serving:

Calories   360
% Daily Value*
Total Fat 11.2g   14%
Saturated Fat 2.6g   13%
Cholesterol 9mg   3%
Sodium 305mg   13%
Total Carbohydrate 60.2g 22%
Dietary Fiber 2.1g   8%
Total Sugars 45.2g
Protein 9g

Directions:
1. Mix the broken whole wheat biscuits and almond butter in a bowl.
2. Press this biscuit mixture firmly onto the base of a spring form pan or individual serving plates to create a uniform layer.
3. Combine the low-fat ricotta cheese, Greek yogurt, and honey in a separate mixing dish. Blend it well.
4. Transfer the cheesecake filling mixture onto the biscuit base in the pan or plates, ensuring even distribution using a spatula.
5. Refrigerate the cheesecake for at least 2-3 hours.
6. Top it with a variety of berries and jelly pieces.
7. Serve and savor.

CHAPTER 10:

DRINK & SMOOTHIES

Green Detox Smoothie

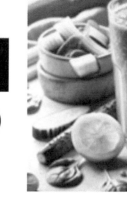

Ingredients:

- 2 cups fresh spinach leaves
- 2 green apples, cored and chopped
- 1/2 cucumber, peeled and diced
- 2 celery stalks, chopped
- juice of 1 lemon
- 1-1/4 cup coconut water

Simple | 5 minutes | 2

0 minutes | 5 minutes

Nutritional Values per Serving:

Calories 159
% Daily Value*
Total Fat 1g 1%
Saturated Fat 0.1g 1%
Cholesterol 0mg 0%
Sodium 162mg 7%
Total Carbohydrate 38.3g 14%
Dietary Fiber 9.3g 33%
Total Sugars 25.4g
Protein 4.3g

Directions:

1. First, wash all the vegetables and fruit properly.
2. Take a high-speed blender and add the spinach leaves, green apple, cucumber, celery stalks, and lemon juice. At the end, add the coconut water.
3. Add ice cubes for chilling.
4. Pulse the ingredients at high speed for 1 minute until smooth in consistency.
5. Pour the green Detox smoothie into ice-filled serving glasses.
6. Serve and enjoy immediately.

Cucumber and Mint Flavored Water

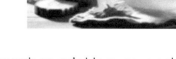

Ingredients:

- 1 cucumber, thinly sliced
- handful of fresh mint leaves
- 1 lemon, thinly sliced
- 4 cups sparkling water, chilled

Simple | 10 minutes | 2

0 minutes | 10 minutes

Nutritional Values per Serving:

Calories   22
% Daily Value*
Total Fat 0.2g 0%
Saturated Fat 0g   0%
Cholesterol 0mg   0%
Sodium 4mg 0%
Total Carbohydrate 6.5g   2%
Dietary Fiber 1.7g   6%
Total Sugars 2.1g
Protein 0.9g

Directions:

1. Start by properly washing the cucumber, mint leaves, and lemon under cold water.
2. Slice the cucumber and lemon into thin cuts, usually round.
3. Tear and slightly crush the mint leaves gently to release the aroma. Add the sliced cucumber, mint leaves, and lemon slices in a large pitcher.
4. Pour sparkling water on top of it, ensuring all the ingredients are submerged.
5. Stir well and let it not distribute so the flavors are infused evenly.
6. Let it sit in the refrigerator for at least 30 minutes or longer for better taste.
7. When ready to serve, fill glasses with ice cubes and pour them.
8. Enjoy

Peach Iced Tea

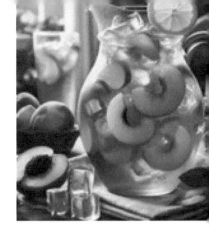

Ingredients:
- 4 black tea bags
- 2 ripe peaches, pitted and sliced
- 1/3 cup honey (adjust to taste)
- 2 lemons, juice only
- 6 cups water

 Simple 10 minutes 2

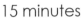 5 minutes · 15 minutes

Nutritional Values per Serving:
Calories 112
% Daily Value*
Total Fat 0.4g 1%
Saturated Fat 0g 0%
Cholesterol 0mg 0%
Sodium 28mg 1%
Total Carbohydrate 28.3g 10%
Dietary Fiber 2.3g 8%
Total Sugars 27.7g
Protein 1.5g

Directions:
1. Take a large saucepan and boil water for about 6 cups.
2. Put the tea bags in the saucepan and let it steep for a few minutes.
3. Then, discard the tea bags.
4. Add the sliced peaches to the hot tea and allow them to steep for 10-15 minutes, infusing it well.
5. Next, gently blend in the honey and stir so it dissolves.
6. Juice the juice from 2 lemons into the tea, stirring for a fine combination.
7. Let it cool to room temperature, and then transfer it into a pitcher.
8. Place the pitcher in the refrigerator and chill for 1-2 hours.
9. Serve once ready.

Chia Berry and Seed Smoothie

Ingredients:
- 1 cup of blueberries
- ½ cup of raspberries
- 1 teaspoon of chia seeds
- 1/3 cup of low-fat greek yogurt
- ¼ cup of low-fat almond milk

 Simple 5 minutes 1

 5 minutes · 5 minutes

Nutritional Values per Serving:
Calories 255
% Daily Value*
Total Fat 16.3g 21%
Saturated Fat 12.7g 63%
Cholesterol 0mg 0%
Sodium 10mg 0%
Total Carbohydrate 26.4g 10%
Dietary Fiber 7g 25%
Total Sugars 14.1g
Protein 4.7g

Directions:
1. Take a high-speed blender and add all the ingredients listed.
2. Pulse it on high for 30 -60 seconds.
3. Pour the smoothie into tall ice-filled serving glasses.
4. Serve it chilled, and enjoy

Lavender Lemonade

Ingredients:

- 2 cups water
- 1 lemon, juice
- 2 teaspoons of dried/ fresh lavender
- 1 teaspoon of honey
-

 Simple 10 minutes 1

 5 minutes 15 minutes

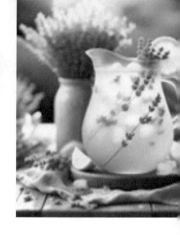

Nutritional Values per Serving:

Calories 93
% Daily Value*
Total Fat 0.3g 0%
Saturated Fat 0g 0%
Cholesterol 0mg 0%
Sodium 9mg 0%
Total Carbohydrate 26.6g 10%
Dietary Fiber 2.8g 10%
Total Sugars 19.8g
Protein 1.2g

Directions:

1. Take a saucepan and add water to the boiling
2. Once simmering, add lavender and turn off the flame.
3. Let the lavender steep for 30 minutes in water.
4. Add honey and stir well so it dissolves in water.
5. Once cool, add lemon juice and let it chill in the refrigerator for at least 1-2 hours to allow the flavors to meld and the drink to cool.
6. When it's ready to serve, fill the glasses with ice cubes and pour the chilled lavender lemonade over the ice.
7. Serve and enjoy.

Banana & Peanut Butter Milkshake

Ingredients:

- 2 frozen bananas, peeled
- 1 tablespoon of natural peanut butter
- ¼ cup of almond milk
- ice cubes for chilling

 Simple 5 minutes 1

0 minutes 5 minutes

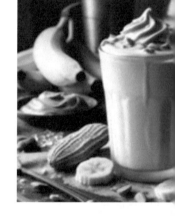

Nutritional Values per Serving:

Calories 159
% Daily Value*
Total Fat 14g 18%
Saturated Fat 6.8g 34%
Cholesterol 0mg 0%
Sodium 10mg 0%
Total Carbohydrate 4.9g 2%
Dietary Fiber 1.6g 6%
Total Sugars 2.1g
Protein 5.6g

Directions:

1. Take a high-speed blender and add frozen bananas to it
2. Add natural peanut butter along with almond milk and ice cubes
3. Pulse the blender for 1 minute until smooth.
4. Put some more almond milk, depending on your desired thickness.
5. Taste the milkshake and adjust the taste by adding more peanut butter
6. Pour it into tall serving glasses, serve it chilled, and enjoy.

Tropical Smoothie

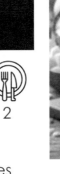

Ingredients:

- 1 cup mango, pulp
- ½ cup of pineapple chunks
- 2 frozen and peeled bananas, cubed
- ½ cup of coconut water
- ice cubes for chilling

Simple   10 minutes   2
0 minutes   10 minutes

Directions:

1. Take a high-speed blender and add all the listed ingredients to it
2. Pulse at high for 1 minute
3. Pour into tall ice-filled glasses and serve.

Nutritional Values per Serving:

Calories 159
% Daily Value*
Total Fat 0.7g 1%
Saturated Fat 0.3g 1%
Cholesterol 0mg 0%
Sodium 66mg 3%
Total Carbohydrate 40g 15%
Dietary Fiber 4.9g 17%
Total Sugars 25.3g
Protein 2.3g

Lemon and Strawberry Infused Water

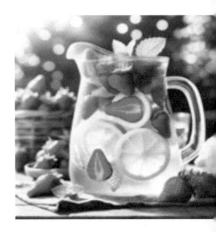

Ingredients:

- 2 cups strawberries, sliced
- 1 lemon, sliced
- 5-6 fresh mint leaves
- 8 cups water

Simple   10 minutes   2
0 minutes   10 minutes

Directions:

1. The first step is to wash the strawberries, lemon, and mint leaves well.
2. Hull the strawberries and then slice them roundly.
3. Next, cut the lemon into thin rounds and remove all the seeds.
4. Combine the sliced strawberries, lemon rounds, and a few sprigs of fresh mint leaves in a large pitcher.
5. Pour water into the pitcher, ensuring that all the ingredients are submerged.
6. Stir and cover the pitcher and refrigerate for at least 2 hours.
7. Serve it chilled.

Nutritional Values per Serving:

Calories 43
% Daily Value*
Total Fat 0.5g 1%
Saturated Fat 0.1g 0%
Cholesterol 0mg 0%
Sodium 22mg 1%
Total Carbohydrate 10.9g 4%
Dietary Fiber 4.3g 16%
Total Sugars 3.7g
Protein 1.8g

Mango Smoothie

Ingredients:

- 2 ripe mangoes, peeled and pitted
- 1 cup greek yogurt
- 1/2 teaspoon ground cardamom
- 1/2 tablespoon stevia
- 1 cup cold water

Simple   5 minutes   2

0 minutes   5 minutes

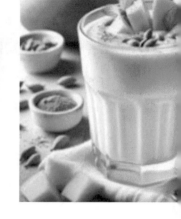

Nutritional Values per Serving:

Calories 162
% Daily Value*
Total Fal 1.4g 2%
Saturated Fat 0.9g 4%
Cholesterol 3mg 1%
Sodium 20mg 1%
Total Carbohydrate 34.3g 12%
Dietary Fiber 1.6g 6%
Total Sugars 32.9g
Protein 5.9g

Directions:

1. Combine the mango chunks, Greek yogurt, ground cardamom, honey, and cold water with a high-speed blender.
2. Blend on high speed until smooth.
3. Serve immediately and enjoy the exotic and refreshing flavors of this mango smoothie.

Pomegranate Antioxidant Smoothie

Ingredients:

- 1 cup pomegranate seeds
- 1 cup blueberries
- 2 ripe bananas, frozen and peeled
- 1 cup greek yogurt
- 1/4 cup water

Simple   5 minutes   2

0 minutes   5 minutes

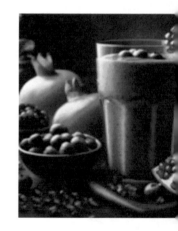

Nutritional Values per Serving:

Calories 191
% Daily Value*
Total Fat 1.5g 2%
Saturated Fat 0.9g 4%
Cholesterol 3mg 1%
Sodium 18mg 1%
Total Carbohydrate 40.7g 15%
Dietary Fiber 4.2g 15%
Total Sugars 23.5g
Protein 6.9g

Directions:

1. Put all the ingredients in a high-speed blender.
2. Pulse the ingredients at a high speed until smooth and creamy.
3. Pour more water to achieve the desired consistency if the smoothie is thick.
4. Serve and enjoy.

Conclusion

In conclusion, the DASH diet is a powerful tool for improving overall health and controlling high blood pressure. It surely provides a well-balanced eating protocol by emphasizing fiber-rich foods like fruits, rich and whole vegetables, nuts, lean proteins, whole grains, and low-fat dairy products.

Moreover, it not only helps lower blood pressure but also helps with weight loss, heart health, and overall fitness.

In this book, we easily explain and cover all the basic principles of the DASH diet, exploring its origins, scientific evidence, and practical application.

We provided precise information about the DASH diet's health benefits, its effectiveness in reducing blood pressure, lowering cholesterol levels, and eliminating the risk of chronic illnesses such as kideny disease, heart failure, stroke, and type 2 diabetes.

Moreover, we've offered a variety of delicious and nutritious recipes that showcase the diverse range of foods that can be enjoyed while following the DASH diet so that the overall transition goes smoothly.

From hearty snacks to smoothies to satisfying main courses and delectable desserts, our recipes demonstrate that eating healthily can be both delicious and satisfying.

As you embark on your journey to adopt the DASH diet, remember that small changes can dramatically improve your health over time. Whether you want to lose blood pressure, improve cholesterol, or adopt a healthier lifestyle, the DASH diet offers a simple and sustainable way to eat that can help everyone.

By adopting the core principles of the DASH diet into your daily life and making informed meal choices, you can take control of your health and achieve lifelong vitality and well-being. Here's to your health and happiness on your DASH food journey.

Bonus 1 Meel Plan_____

BONUS 2 Shopping list + Brief Overview

Bonus 3 Smart Replacement for Celiac_____

Bonus 4 Complementary Physical Activity

14+14 NUTRIFIT METHOD

REFERENCES

[1] Miller, M. D., & Appel, L. J. (2023). The DASH Diet for the prevention and treatment of hypertension. Journal of Clinical Hypertension (Greenwich), 25(9), 1422-1431.

[2] Mente, A., de Lorgeril, M., & O'Donnell, M. (2020). Dietary approaches to stop hypertension (DASH) for blood pressure and cardiovascular risk reduction: A comprehensive review and meta-analysis. European Journal of Preventive Cardiology, 27(1), 1-11.Sacks, F. M., Svetkey,

[3] L. P., Vollmer, W. M., Dawson, C., & Bernstein, L. (2001). Effects on blood pressure of sodium reduction with the DASH Diet compared to an American Heart Association-recommended diet. Journal of the American Medical Association, 286(2), 289-298.

[4] National Kidney Foundation. (2023). Stages of chronic kidney disease (CKD).

[5] Grandner, M. A., Troyer, M. L., & Allison, P. (2017). The short-sleep paradox in healthy adults: Why sleep quantity is important but insufficient for optimal health. Sleep Health, 3(4), 301-310.

[6] National Heart, Lung, and Blood Institute. (2023). DASH Eating Plan - Dietary Approaches to Stop Hypertension.

[7] Appel, L. J., & Sacks, F. M. (2009). The DASH Diet and its potential benefits for diabetes mellitus. Journal of Clinical Hypertension (Greenwich), 11(1), 6-11.

[8] Burke, L. M., & Deakin, V. (2010). Sport nutrition and performance. Human Kinetics.

[9] National Kidney Foundation. (2023, January). Stages of chronic kidney disease (CKD)

[10] Prewitt, R. C., & Tangney, C. C. (2017). DASH Diet for blood pressure and weight management. The New England Journal of Medicine, 376(9), 856-864.

[11] American Heart Association. (2023). Cholesterol.

[12] American College of Obstetricians and Gynecologists. (2023). High blood pressure during pregnancy.

[13] Mensink, R.P., et al., Effects of dietary fatty acids and carbohydrates on the ratio of serum total to HDL cholesterol and on serum lipids and apolipoproteins: a meta-analysis of 60 controlled trials. Am J Clin Nutr, 2003. 77(5): p. 1146-55.

[14] U.S. Department of Agriculture, U.S.D.o.H.a.H.S., Washington, D.C.: U.S. Government Printing Office. Dietary Guidelines for Americarewrns, 2010, 2010.

[15] Lichtenstein, A.H., et al., Diet and lifestyle recommendations revision 2006: a scientific statement from the American Heart Association Nutrition Committee. Circulation, 2006. 114(1): p. 82-96.

16. Siri-Tarino, P.W., et al., Meta-analysis of prospective cohort studies evaluating the association of saturated fat with cardiovascular disease. Am J Clin Nutr, 2010. 91(3): p. 535-46.

[17]. Micha, R. and D. Mozaffarian, Saturated fat and cardiometabolic risk factors, coronary heart disease, stroke, and diabetes: a fresh look at the evidence. Lipids, 2010. 45(10): p. 893-905.

[18]. https://www.ncbi.nlm.nih.gov/pmc/articles/PMC7019370/

[19]. https://pubmed.ncbi.nlm.nih.gov/26503843/

[20]. https://pubmed.ncbi.nlm.nih.gov/32735225/

[21] "The science behind the DASH Eating Plan | NHLBI, NIH," NHLBI, NIH. https://www.nhlbi.nih.gov/education/dash/research#:~:text=Reducing%20daily%20sodium%20lowered%20blood,with%20each%20reduction%20of%20sodium

[22] M. J. Belanger et al., "Effects of the dietary approaches to stop hypertension diet on change in cardiac biomarkers over time: results from the DASH-Sodium trial," Journal of the American Heart Association, vol. 12, no. 2, Jan. 2023, doi: 10.1161/jaha.122.026684.

[23] T. J. Moore, P. R. Conlin, J. D. Ard, and L. P. Svetkey, "DASH (Dietary Approaches to Stop Hypertension) diet is effective treatment for Stage 1 isolated systolic hypertension," Hypertension, vol. 38, no. 2, pp. 155–158, Aug. 2001, doi: 10.1161/01.hyp.38.2.155.

[24] S. P. Juraschek, M. Woodward, F. M. Sacks, V. J. Carey, E. R. Miller, and L. J. Appel, "Time course of change in blood pressure from sodium reduction and the DASH Diet," Hypertension, vol. 70, no. 5, pp. 923–929, Nov. 2017, doi: 10.1161/hypertensionaha.117.10017.

Made in the USA
Columbia, SC
04 September 2024

41373601R00043